Practice made Perfect: Higher level aspirations for practice nurses

Practice made Perfect: Higher level aspirations for practice nurses

Hilary Paniagua

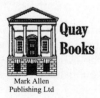

Quay Books

Mark Allen
Publishing Ltd

Quay Books Division, Mark Allen Publishing Limited
Jesses Farm, Snow Hill, Dinton, Wiltshire, SP3 5HN

British Library Cataloguing-in-Publication Data
A catalogue record is available for this book

© Mark Allen Publishing Ltd 2001
ISBN 1 85642 173 2

Printed in the UK by The Bath Press, Bath

Contents

Preface

Hilary Paniagua's seminal text on advancing practice is timely for a number of reasons. First, she has provided a comprehensive contextual picture of the contemporary developments of the practice nurse role. Second, she has been able to pitch this development into the important realms of advanced practice with reasoned arguments of why practice nurses should aspire to this level of practice. Finally, she has been able to articulate a vision for the future for practice nurse development at an advanced level that is both realistic and far-sighted in realising the undoubted potential of practice nurses. Hawkins (2000) notes that nurses referred to their patients,

...listened to their needs and created care to meet those needs. What distinguished nurses from other providers was their presence.

Practice nurses have these attributes in spades. They are in the right place at the right time for patients. What better reason could they possibly have than this for advancing their practice to really make a difference?

Roswyn Hakesley-Brown
Mphil, BA, RN, RM, DN (Lond) RNT, Cert Ed (Bham)
Independent Consultant in Health Care Education
President of the Royal College of Nursing

Introduction

Practice nursing is in a state of dynamic change; scope now exists for nurses to move forward in their careers and there is an exciting future ahead for those who have vision and enthusiasm for change. Opportunities to progress have led nurses in search of new knowledge and skills in order to realise their vision and provide more proficient, holistic and innovative care. They are becoming experts in their field and practising with considerable 'know how' and ability. Such expertise and aptitude is recognised within advanced practice and the role of the advanced nurse practitioner (ANP). ANPs earn their reputation by excelling in critical judgement ability and demonstrating high levels of interpersonal skills and mastery of care.

However, historically this role has not been without its difficulties, as confusion exists over the title and what actually constitutes advanced practice. This book provides some possible answers and recognises that there will always be a call for experts within nursing and that the role of the ANP will forever be a reality, despite professional change and agitation.

This expert role is not straightforward and those preparing for it require a source of reference and background understanding to equip themselves with the knowledge and scope of skills required. This book aims to contribute to that and provide practice nurses with fresh insights into some of the issues surrounding the role of the ANP. It also hopes to offer suggestions as to how advanced practice can be incorporated into the field of general practice, focusing on the function and specific knowledge involved. The content is also appropriate for practice nurses who may not yet want to become ANPs, but wish to gain more knowledge of specialist and professional issues or just acquire new skills. The potential for all to learn from this book will also make it useful to nurse practitioners and nurses aspiring to become specialists.

Undergraduates, post-graduate students, teachers and all practice nurses should find this book useful as a reference to expert practice. Every effort was taken to devise this as a complete text on the role of ANP, and while aimed at general practice, the general concepts of advanced practice can be transferred to any speciality. Each chapter can therefore be viewed separately, and be of use in dealing with individual issues or relevant knowledge required. Inevitably, by the time a book is published there may be issues within professional life that have moved on. Every attempt has been made to ensure that the content of all chapters are up-to-date and professionally relevant.

It is hoped that this book will help to develop the skills and knowledge of every practice nurse and particularly those wishing to acquire expert roles. It aims to show all nurses the way to make valuable contributions to the clients they serve and how to pave the way to advance the profession of nursing as a whole.

1

The historical development of advanced nursing practice within general practice

*All professions are conspiracies against
the laity.*

George Bernard Shaw

The role of the practice nurse has witnessed a rebirth over the past few years, and the factors influencing this change remain debatable. Policy imperatives have a large part to play in shaping the destiny of practice nursing. There is little doubt, however, that individual career aspirations and the need for practice nursing to prove itself as a credible discipline has contributed to its new professional identity and legitimacy. The path has not been a smooth one and it could be the case that its direction has evolved more from a knee-jerk reaction to facilitating contractual arrangements for general practitioner (GP) services than from deliberate design. The end result clearly justifies the response as practice nursing, a role once conceived of as only for the GP's wife (Damant *et al*, 1994), has now become a credible position where some nurses work pro-actively as autonomous practitioners in their own right (Hardy, 1995).

While the foundations of practice nursing were being set, parallel developments were taking place in the United States. The notion of the nurse practitioner (NP) began to evolve with its roots embedded in the concepts of direct care assessor and provider. This image of an autonomous practitioner, who patients chose to consult, sat easily within the realms of general practice and shared close similarities with the characteristics of practice nursing. The background was there for enlightened GPs to encourage and support nurses into expanding their roles and take on increased responsibility and develop more skills, and nurses began to develop under the characteristics of NPs in work, if not in title. Touché Ross (1994) highlights that NPs working in general practice managing a comprehensive list of patients now have the clearest caseload and highest workload.

The scenario is still unfolding for practice nurses, as society, political forces and professional pressures are looking for this discipline to go one step further. Practice nurses now take the place of retired GPs, become GP partners or become pioneers of primary care pilot schemes. Practice nurses have been given the opportunity to show their worth and gradually the nursing world, together with the general public, are beginning to see value in practice nursing. The real challenge now is to lead community nursing through the new Millennium, and this potential lies within the capacity of the advanced nurse practitioner (ANP). The actual definition and avenues of this role are explained in the following chapter and it can be seen to have many commonalties with both the NP and practice nurse role (*Table 1.1*).

While the level of practice is recognised, the name of the ANP may change to suit the capriciousness of the United Kingdom Central Council for Nursing and Midwifery who have launched yet another round of pilot scheme consultations to determine higher levels of practice (UKCC, 1998). Those who look to the UKCC for their destiny, however, may be disappointed, as Walsh (1999) pictures the UKCC as already shipwrecked on a reef of its own making. However, the restructuring that is in progress at this time of writing to replace it with the Nursing and Midwifery Council in the near future, may bring about a more enlightened approach to regulation at different levels.

The future can only be charted by understanding how the past has led up to the present, and for practice nurses this history, while comprehensive, takes place over a relatively short time span.

The developing role of the nurse in general practice

In the 1960s it was unusual for nurses to work alongside GPs, and for those that did, little information existed about their work and little is known about practice nurses employed during this time. Nursing care was undertaken mainly in the patient's home by district nurses. For the few patients who were mobile, some health authorities attached specific district nurses to work within surgeries. The role developed through undertaking agreed surgery treatments and patient referrals received from GPs during surgery times. It was during the 1960s that family practitioner committees decided to reimburse GPs with 70% of the salary costs of two non-medical staff, which included nurses. This provided an incentive to employ nurses which must have been hard to resist for GPs, particularly as there was much publicity in GP journals explaining how nurses could be of

Table 1.1: Role commonalities

	Advanced nurse practitioner in general practice	Specialist practitioner	Nurse practitioner	Practice nurse
Access	Provides direct access for patients and has recognised credibility as an expert in a specialist field.	Provides direct access for patients over a broad area of problems.	Provides direct access for patients over a broad area of problems, although mostly acute.	Provides direct access for patients over a broad range of acute and chronic conditions. May also have specialist responsibilities in asthma or diabetes management.
Range of autonomy	Acts autonomously, able to take on in-depth patient management and chosen sub-roles. Utilises and develops protocols.	Acts autonomously in management of clients, utilising and devising protocols.	Acts autonomously in management of clients, incorporating the use of protocols.	Acts autonomously in management of clients, utilising and devising protocols.
Level of client assessment	Assesses the health of client holistically, utilising physical examination skills, expert knowledge and high level of critical thinking ability. Assessment based on relationship built over time with patients, and knowledge of their families and backgrounds. Underpinned by mastery of thought and high level of thinking and experiential knowledge. Academic ability underpinned by a Masters degree.	Assess the health of clients using history-taking and possible examination abilities. Able to assess from a relationship underpinned by knowledge of patients, their families and environment. Critical thinking and academic ability at degree level.	Assesses the health of clients using history-taking and physical examination. Academic ability ranges from diploma to Masters level.	Assesses the health of clients, using history-taking and limited physical examination abilities. Able to assess from a relationship underpinned through knowledge of patient's family background and environment. Training and academic ability varies, mostly in-house training, short courses and attendance on study days.
Range of referral	Refers patients to physicians and a broad scope of other agencies, knowledge of which is gained through networking and other professional activities.	Refers patients to other agencies. Referral to physicians rare but possible.	Refers patients to physicians and other agencies.	Refers patients to other nursing agencies.
Role components	Utilises characteristics of leadership, collaborator, change agent, innovator, research, manager, role model and teacher. These sub-roles may or may not be utilised altogether, however, whatever is used, great prominence and creativity is shown in response to needs of the health care of patients and nursing as a profession. Leadership may take the form of primary care group (PCG) board member or chairperson. Probable instigator of pilot scheme.	Roles differ according to personal incentive and opportunities. Will contribute to or undertake audit. May also take leadership role on PCG boards. Adapts the sub-roles of teacher, leader and researcher.	Normally only utilises clinical components of role, although may contribute to research and teaching others.	Will contribute to or undertake audit and research. May also take leadership role on PCG boards.

financial benefit by performing fee-for-service tasks (eg. cervical smears and immunisations/vaccinations), tasks for which GPs received extra payments. The money generated from this in itself would have paid for the 30% salary deficit.

Perhaps unwittingly there was a general lure to employ practice nurses and a small number of nurses, known as facilitators, began to be employed in health authorities. Their remit was to put pressure on GPs to work with nurses to undertake preventative health care, such as screening clinics for coronary heart disease and stroke prevention.

Not surprisingly, there was a steady increase in the number of privately-employed practice nurses around this time, although very little is known about their work. Most of the early investigations into practice nurse roles were undertaken by Reedy (1972) and Bowling (1981), which uncovered mainly the clinical treatment tasks performed, such as blood pressure monitoring, venepuncture and smear-taking. In fact, Reedy (1972) identified a total of 45 tasks to be found in various surgeries across the country. Much of the literature remained anecdotal or mere descriptions of common nursing tasks, and this did not take into account the extent, variation and nature of practice nurse work.

Studies were limited in identifying the role of practice nurses as agents of first contact, listeners, advisers and facilitators of health education and promotion. Practice nurses were quietly increasing the breadth of their role through the years, unhindered by the bureaucracy of a nursing hierarchy and unnoticed by other nursing disciplines and powers. The potential for role development was timely and nurses began to develop more autonomous roles such as Barbara Stillwell, whose work earned her the reputation of being the first NP in Britain.

The vast increase in practice nurse employment by GPs, together with the freedom to experiment with their roles, caused an undercurrent of unease in the nursing world. Concerns developed over task transference from GPs to nurses and there were calls to control delegation. There was widespread confusion over appropriate roles and the legal situation, and there were differences in opinion within districts and surgeries, particularly in the case of health authority-employed district nurses still doing surgery sessions.

The Royal College of Nursing (RCN) and the Royal College of General Practitioners (RCGP) were forced to issue a report (RCN and RCGP, 1974) stating that there were no statutory regulations on what a nurse can or cannot do. However, the Department of Health and Social Security (DHSS, 1997) recommended that any delegation should take place within clearly defined policy at local levels.

Such policies related only to health authority-employed practice nurses, not to GP-employed practice nurses who continued to practice independently. The background was set for potential resentment and jealously against practice nurses by those in the nursing professions who saw them as a threat and were unable to comprehend any practice beyond the traditional boundaries. Such feelings did little to endear practice nurses with their fellow community colleagues.

The debate and any animosity came to a head with the *Cumberledge Report on Community Nursing* (DHSS, 1986). Under the auspices of investigating the quality, efficiency and cost-effectiveness of community nursing, the Cumberledge Review Body recommended that GPs no longer be reimbursed for the salary of practice nurses as this led to a fragmented workforce. It is of little surprise to the more cynical that the report suggested that funds should be transferred to the community nursing service budget, so that the health authority could employ, allocate and manage practice nurses. It made no provision, however, for priority to be given to keep the posts already occupied by practice nurses. There was also a general dissatisfaction with the credibility of such nurses, which stemmed principally from criticism of poor practice nurse training which had been mainly carried out in-house by GPs.

The need to stop reimbursement was further justified by claims that it was unfair for the National Health Service (NHS) to, in effect, pay twice by virtue of salary and fee-for-service tasks. This would have resulted in the phasing out of practice nurses employed by GPs, a loss of 4000 jobs. The report went on further to recommend the implementation of NPs based on the USA model, and while it failed to clarify whether practice nurses would be suitable, it clearly saw suitability within the district nurses' role and training.

The RCN sympathised with the report's recommendations in curtailing reimbursement and in phasing out GP employed nurses. Little thought was given to protecting jobs and practice nurses were faced with potential unemployment. There was no guarantee that health authorities would see value in their role as distinct from district nursing or indeed employ them.

Inevitably these moves angered many practice nurses and GPs, although with GPs, how much of their motives stemmed from the threat of losing financial benefits rather than preventing unemployment for colleagues, must be debatable. Threatened practice nurses fought hard to make their voices heard, supported by reports to the Government by the General Medical Services Committee

(1986) who reacted negatively to phasing out reimbursements for staff. Many nurses, disillusioned with the RCN, sought an alternative defence body within the Medical Defence Union, and this still remains a viable option, if not first choice for some practice nurses today. After many battles and reports, the DHSS finally rejected the Cumberledge Team's recommendations for changes to the employment structure of practice nurses and the abolition of fee-for-service fees. This heralded the emergence of practice nursing as a credible discipline, and is a testimony to their drive and instincts to fight for their deserved recognition. Also, the professional and supportive relationship with GPs should not be underestimated or forgotten, as the dispute was not fought alone.

The changing face of practice nursing

While some disciplines remained entrenched in routine and task-centred approaches to care, practice nurses were now free to develop their roles. Implicit to this role was the specific emphasis on health promotion. Concern began to develop that the responsibilities of community nurses were being eroded by practice nurses, particularly heath visitors who saw themselves as having a dedicated role in prevention (Williams and Sibbald, 1999). Practice nurse emphasis on prevention, while worthwhile, was mainly the result of the Government's new political culture where prevention was seen to be cheaper than cure. The governmental philosophy of promoting health and preventing disease was pledged in White Papers such as *Promoting Better Health* (DoH, 1987) and *Working for Patients* (DoH, 1989a), all of which impinged upon the responsibility of GPs and the workload of practice nurses. The 1990 *GP Contract* (DoH, 1989b) saw the culmination of health promotion targets as a formally recognised part of GP services, and contract opportunities arose for which the experience of practice nurses in promotional activities provided the momentum. Payment was given to surgeries based on the uptake of the services offered, substantiated with evidence of efficient data collection. While practice nurses helped GPs to meet their contractual obligations, GPs were able to concentrate more on their management and financial earnings or use nurses as a realistic strategy to generate savings in their time.

Among areas eligible for financial entitlements were minor surgery, reaching the uptake of 90% of childhood immunisations and

80% of cervical smears, yearly visits to the over 75s, new patient registration checks, child health surveillance and health promotion clinics. As a consequence of these incentives, practice nurses found themselves performing home visits to perform elderly assessment. This practice did little to impress their district nursing colleagues and enhance working relationships. Concerns also arose that practice nurses did not have the appropriate training to undertake their new roles. However, despite lack of academic backing, practice nurses began to establish working groups to develop in-house training, sponsored by drug companies and supported by practice nurse facilitators by offering study days and workshops. There was no limit to the enterprising capabilities of practice nurses in their quest for training. However, because this did not involve formal academic creditation or courses equivalent to other community colleagues, practice nurses appeared to be viewed as the poor relations in the nursing world, with no recognised credibility for the pro-active work they undertook.

Roles began to develop in working alongside GPs in innovative health promotion clinics. Many nurses helped to devise the necessary protocols and some ran the clinics by themselves, depending on their areas of expertise. There were no restrictions placed on GPs to control the area or content of such clinics, and many nurses working at this time will remember the prolifications of approaches to health promotion from exercise to stress reduction sessions. There were many cynical comments at this time about the dubious nature of some clinics run in the name of health promotion, such as dog walking.

Practices could run up to eight clinics per month, for which they received a payment incentive of £30 per clinic, given that they could prove attendance of a minimum of 10 patients per clinic. The impetus to find enough patients each month to attend sessions gradually declined, as did the hectic workload of practice nurses, forced to run clinics on top of their own surgery sessions. In the following year, GPs were able to claim for their specific promotional activities if patients were seen in the course of their daily consultations, and not necessarily in specified clinics, and the pressure was lessened.

As a result of the previous open approach to clinics and perhaps some notion of the potential for some GPs to take advantage, in 1993 the Government introduced a new system of payments. The Family Health Service Authority (once known as Family Practitioner Committees) became more formally involved in the GP targets and remunerative clinics. The aim was to focus interventions onto more defined priority groups, such as those at risk due to smoking, coronary heart disease (CHD) and stroke. Payment was again based on the uptake of services and the submission of data within three proposed bands.

Practices were eligible to apply for the band criteria they felt they could accommodate best. Band 1 was for practices thought only wanting to offer smoking cessation activities. Band 2 centred around reducing the morbidity and mortality in CHD and stroke. Band 3 offered the most payment and therefore the most work and included the activities within the other two bands, plus now offering, instead of requiring, annual home visits to the over 75s and health promotion consultations to new patients. Predictably, most practices applied for Band 3 status.

The change in working brought with it fears for change within practice nursing. The key difference now was a reduction in clinic work combined with the fact that elderly assessment and new patient medicals were no longer a compulsory service. No doubt, responsibility for this shift lay to some extent in the fact that some over 75s resented health checks as an intrusion into their independent lives and homes, and patients who moved surgeries could not understand why they needed a medical check when they were perfectly healthy the day before in their previous surgery.

It seemed very likely that practice nurses would find themselves redundant, particularly newer ones employed predominantly to run health promotion clinics. Rumours of unemployment began to hit the nursing press, however, it seems practice nurses had become too valuable to lose, as they were still needed as key players because of their knowledge of audit and computers. Hence, the growth in practice nursing that had arisen out of political impulse in the past was set to remain under its system of the future. The number of practice nurses in England and Wales employed as a result of contractual arrangements was estimated to be approximately 13,500 whole-time equivalent nurses in 1992.

Practice nurse survival owed much to the flexibility and ability to prove their worth alongside GPs in providing quality and efficiency in primary care. The timing of this had also been opportune, as it coincided with the introduction of a competitive and internal market ethos within the NHS. Practice nurses were now recognised as crucial players in general practice, providing greater consumer choice as first levels of contact. The convenience of having practice nurses guaranteed many GPs the prominent places they were seeking in the powerful primary care market of fund-holding, where there was a reversal of power relationships between hospitals and primary care. The White Paper, *Working for Patients* (DoH, 1989a) had installed an internal market giving GPs a high status as guardians of commissioning as well as providers of health care services. Many GPs now spent time in pursuing their own agenda and the perceived demands of their new role. Relentless pressure on GPs by policy makers improved the status of practice nurses considerably as they became the essential workforce in taking much of the clinical workload off overburdened GPs. As GPs had greater freedom to run their surgeries, develop services and chase contracts, practice nurses provided the core support and a blueprint for practice, which would ensure growth opportunities in terms of money, competition and innovation.

This period saw radical change in service provision from the secondary sector to primary care, and GP surgeries began to take on board the work of endoscopies, sigmoidoscopies, scanning and extensive minor surgery, all of which needed practice nurse input in organisation and nursing care. Practice nurses began to develop skills in facilitating minor surgery and the necessary care of patients receiving it.

GPs were beginning to offer comprehensive services within the community; the control and provision of which held much financial appeal in savings and profit. Fund-holding gave GPs the advantage of altering the mix of expenditure and opportunities for carrying savings over from one year to the next. Practice nurses proved helpful in financial initiatives, particularly in April 1993, when fund-holding was extended to cover the purchase of community nursing, which meant not only more influence over monetary control but also potential authority over nursing employment.

In the practices that took over the community-nursing budget, numerous practice nurses found themselves as managers of primary health care teams and thus team leaders in primary care. The entrepreneurial skills of practice nurses allowed GPs to compete successfully within the market and in return nurses gained a wealth of experience including that of running integrated nursing teams. Practice nurse knowledge was underpinned by a career structure in strategic management, professional collaboration and developing nursing care within the pressures of a commercial world.

Practice nursing has evolved into a unique discipline over the years, and crucial to this has been the creative ability to provide an environment which can promote professional development and potential. Most has been achieved as a reaction to the situation nurses found themselves in, combined with deliberate actions designed for the protection and benefits of patients. The emphasis on health promotion and interpersonal relationships with patients and GPs has been the cornerstone of their role and the main distinction of their discipline.

Practice nursing dimensions and dilemmas

While practice nursing has come a long way, this discipline may still not be completely equal in terms of opportunity and power to other community nurses; this is evident in the fact that practice nurses are unable to prescribe. This factor alone is a potential setback to practice nurses wishing to provide holistic care to their clients — an essential aspect of advanced practice. The reason for the exclusion of practice nursing as a category for nurse prescribing is unclear, but must inevitably lie in the past stereotyping of practice nurses by the Government and their advisory bodies as little more than doctors' handmaidens. This view does little to credit the rigorous approach practice nurses have now taken towards education or the success of their work in clinical practice.

Practice nursing was excluded from the onset in the initial plans of the *Cumberledge Report* (DHSS, 1986) to cultivate the possibility of permitting nurses to prescribe independently. The Crown Report (DoH, 1989c) led the Department of Health (DoH, 1989d) to put nurse prescribing later on the agenda, and without the hindsight to consider practice nurses. Under the Medical Products (Prescribing by Nurses etc) Act 1992, only those with the recognised qualification of health visitor or district nurse are eligible for prescribing against a special Nursing Formulary. This has become ironic today, in that in obtaining these qualifications, all community nurses share some of the same modules and the same level of education preparation. The only difference is that the final award given will mean that district nurses and health visitors are eligible to prescribe and others cannot. Following successful pilot schemes there is now a national roll out of health visitors and district nurses in prescribing. Many Community Specialist Degree programmes are also encouraged to develop prescribing training within their timetable, however, precluding practice nurses.

While practice nurses may rightly feel aggrieved by the

situation, it is not made easier by reports that some who do have the privilege to prescribe feel unready to accept the responsibility (May, 1997). Such an analogy makes the reality hard to grasp and it is therefore doubtful as to whose interest it is in for nurses to prescribe, and what has driven the purpose behind nurse prescribing. McCartney *et al* (1999) suggest that while benefits to patient care are true, it is likely that nurse prescribing was a tool used by the Conservative Government to achieve its own ends. They believed that the aim was to show the powerful primary care sector of GPs that privilege could be deregulated away, as a tactic to disguise the shortage of doctors by transferring routine aspects of work, and to save time and money under the creation of the current value-for-money ethos. If this is the case it is little wonder practice nurses did not fit into this political ploy, as their eligibility to prescribe might be seen to be influenced too closely by their allegiance to GP employers. It would not help either in saving time or money as presumably for those visiting the surgery, importance lies in obtaining the prescription in the first place, not in who writes it.

Despite this situation, practice nurses seem optimistic that events will change and perhaps this way of thinking was encouraged by the RCN. Practice nurses were almost promised their support and the potential to prescribe by the RCN in their statement that considered the best way forward was to move towards the extension of prescribing rights for nurses with a specialist practice qualification, and this included district nurses, health visitors and practice nurses. These nurses were thought to have an extremely high level of knowledge and best able to prescribe the most appropriate and clinically effective medicines for their patients (RCN, 1997).

Unfortunately the RCN were not directive in saying what they meant by a specialist practice qualification and this led to much speculation and conjecture. Unease began to be created among many practice nurses, which was now coinciding with moves made earlier by the UKCC to determine standards for specialist practice (UKCC, 1994) and their recommendations that it be underpinned by a degree level programme. The first degree programmes within universities had been set up for community nurses in October 1995, based on 50% theory and 50% practice, within four components: clinical practice, clinical practice leadership, practice development and care and programme management. Specialist practitioners were defined by the UKCC (1995) as exercising: 'higher levels of judgement, discretion and decision-making in clinical care', and able to monitor and improve standards of their care through supervision, clinical audit, skilled professional leadership and the development of research-based practice, teaching and the support of professional colleagues.

It can be seen that the remit for this course has connotations of experience and expertise similar to that of advanced practice and the role of the ANP (*Table 1.1*). The roles are so similar in fact that relationships between the boundaries and individual competencies become very blurred. In order to offer some degree of clarity it is perhaps relevant to understand that the majority view is that specialist practice is at degree level while advanced practice is at masters level, which implies that the latter has a higher capacity for mastery of thought and knowledge behind actions and outcomes. This expertise will automatically create a more advanced level of practice, which may cover a broader field of skills. Practitioners will ultimately exhibit more experiential knowledge and ability to intervene when patients present with problems at the extreme of the response continuum, as well as more complex decision-making skills. It is also envisioned that advanced practice implies more responsibility for being a pioneer and adjusting the boundaries of future practice, the remit of such has implications of political astuteness and being a highly visible practitioner and nursing orator. Attempts to shed further light on what constitutes an ANP are considered in the following chapter.

Those wishing to take on the specialist role, because of the similarities with advanced practice, may find the topics covered in this book particularly helpful to them in trying to improve their knowledge and skills or indeed if they hope to move on into the role of ANP.

There has been pressure imposed on practice nurses for a long time to undergo training and gain equal status with their community nurse colleagues. The degree programme offered practice nurses this standardised training equal to other community disciplines for the first time. However, practice nurses who had undertaken many other courses and university programmes, particularly diplomas and NP courses, felt aggrieved that they had already achieved high levels of practice and education and did not want to jump through more hoops. At the same time there was a general concern that prescribing power would be given to those with a community specialist degree and that this would not recognise those who had much expertise to offer already. Following discussions between representatives of the UKCC the English National Board circulated a position statement (UKCC, 1996). Transitional arrangements were promised for those wishing to use the title 'specialist practitioner', providing nurses had followed a course of four months or more in length relevant to the individual's area of practice, and that their employer was confident that they had the skills and knowledge to practice safely and effectively. This meant that many nurses with the ENB A51 course, which fits within this category and is also viewed as the only recognised qualification for practice nurses, were able to use the title 'specialist practitioner'. This was also subject to their employers being content with this. Achievement of this course was only recorded as obtaining an ENB A51 course and not as being a specialist practitioner. There were four pathways available for other practice nurses:

- a first degree in the ENB specialist practitioner programme
- a Dip/HE in the ENB specialist practice programme
- an ENB A51 course
- an APL (assessment of prior learning) with evidence of certificated learning to match the outcomes of the ENB A51.

Time was of the essence as the transitional arrangements were only designed to be an option for nurses until 31 October 1998. After then, the only way to obtain the use of the specialist title was to undergo a first degree ENB specialist programme.

For many other practice nurses without this course there was a stampede to undertake courses quickly being developed by universities, or to submit portfolios for APL towards the necessary accreditation. The pathway was not smooth as practice nurses began to become confused as to which route to take. They were also confused about the difference between those who could now use the title 'specialist practitioner' by virtue of their A51 award or recognition, and those who were awarded degrees and also hold the qualification of specialist practitioner yet have the ensuing mark of specialist practitioner on the UKCC register. Significantly, many nurses today have a variety of qualifications and use of titles, none of which has made them any nearer to prescribing. There also seems to be injustice, as highlighted previously, in the fact that practice nurses undertake the same degree as their colleagues, yet are not allowed to undertake the prescribing component or the separate course as the others do. While practice nurses may understandably be frustrated about this contentious topic, it may be reconciling to know that the Nurse Prescribing Formulary is very limited, and the items available on prescription would be of little use to much of their work with patients and are available for patients over the counter anyway.

There are benefits of being able to provide a more extended formulary of medication for patients within the practice nurse role, particularly when it is needed quickly, such as in acute asthma attacks or as a vital part of successful family planning or disease management clinics. It would also avoid situations practice nurses regularly find themselves in, of writing the prescription and then having to go to someone else to sign it who may never have seen the patient. Patients have already been recognised as being able to benefit from the use of efficient and effective protocol systems (RCN, 1996). For ANPs in general practice, it is important that they can act autonomously in providing holistic care, and the provision of medication is a vital part of that quality care. It could be seen as a natural sequence if required, following on from the ANPs' skills of physical examination and nursing assessment.

The answer for the administration of medicines must be in the use of written protocols. The *Crown Report* (DoH, 1999) defined a group protocol as being:

> *A specific written instruction for the supply or administration of named medicines in an identified clinical situation. It is drawn up locally by doctors, pharmacists and other appropriate professionals, approved by the employer and advised by the relevant advisory committees. It applies to groups of patients or other service users who may not be individually identified before presentation for treatment.*

Protocols take advantage of the provision in the Medicines Act 1968, which allows a nurse to administer a prescription only medicine, 'in accordance with the directions of an appropriate practitioner'. The law has just changed (O'Connor, 2000) which permits the use of protocols through a patient group directive (PGD). This allows drugs to be given to patients who may not have be individually identified before being seen for treatment. Prior to this amendment nurses undertaking mass immunisation were breaking the law, as it was not clear what constituted a 'direction' from a doctor and if a drug protocol actually constituted a 'prescription'. PGDs must be signed by a senior doctor and pharmacist and authorised by the appropriate primary care trust, primary care group or health authority. When setting up protocols practice nurses need to follow the standards for good practice set by the RCN (1993) (*Table 1.2*).

Table 1.2: Guidelines for the administration of medicines under group protocol (RCN, 1993)

Clear statements should answer the following:

Why:

* the service is being set up, including the aims and objectives behind the protocol?

Who:

* will be providing the service and to whom, and who might be excluded from being treated?
* are the professional groups who have approved this protocol?
* is the person who has authorised its use?

When:

* will this service be received and implemented?
* will the protocol be reviewed?

What:

* procedures will be included?
* resources will be needed?
* clinical procedures will be included?
* training or qualifications will be necessary for the professionals involved?
* will be the unambiguous definition of the clinical condition the protocol applies to, and what will be the criteria under which a patient will be eligible?
* will be the criteria for the dosage and route of the medicine, follow-up treatment, instructions, advice, legal status, possible side-effects or special considerations?
* action will be taken for patients who will be excluded or not wish to be treated?
* arrangements are there for referral of the patient and for referral for medical advice?
* details of treatment records are needed?

How:

* will the protocol be monitored and clinical outcomes evaluated?
* will there be a clear audit trail?

The Crown Report (DoH, 1999) also stresses the importance of following the standards laid down within Appendix A (DoH, 1998c). Practitioners wishing to devise appropriate protocols for the administration of medication need to provide the answers to the questions shown in *Table 1.3*, which takes into account the major principles found in this Appendix.

Table 1.3: Principles of protocol development (RCN, 1993)

Protocols are useful and need not conflict with individualised care, providing the following principles for good practice are evident:
* The purpose of the protocol is explicit
* The protocol is founded upon research
* The protocol is not a replacement for individualised care planning
* A protocol is devised only when there is a need to assist nurses and other health professionals to deal with a complex operational issue
* All those who are required to follow the protocol should be involved in its production ·
* All parties should agree the contents of the protocol
* Any party has the right to seek a review of the protocol at any time
* The protocol should be reviewed regularly and when there is a change of circumstances which may affect its proper utilisation.

The finished protocol/PGD needs to be evidence-based, clear and comprehensive, and built within the framework of national guidelines.

Practice nurses have always needed to supply and administer medication. Anderson (1995) highlights that many NPs are supplying prescription only drugs under protocol schemes and that there is a need to expand prescribing nationally to legitimise this behaviour. Hope may be in the Crown Report (DoH, 1999), which outlines possible extensions to prescribing authority. This report mentions including independent and dependent prescribers, see *Table 1.4*. Given the diversity of their role, practice nurses could have a case for arguing that they fit into either category, which makes the future interesting. Change may also be initiated through the NHS Plan (DoH, 2000) which reinforced recent Government incentives to take forward extending the scope of independent nurse prescribing which will not require primary legislation. In April 2000 the Secretary of State announced £10 million to support a training programme to extend the nurse formulary and help to train more nurses to prescribe a wider range of medicines from an expanded Secretary of States' Nurse Prescribers' Formulary.

It is at present under review as to what all this will mean and as to what this formulary will include. There are a number of options which range from no change, ie. maintaining the status quo, to a radical version of prescribing which could include all general sales list items, pharmacy medicines, all licensed prescription only medicines and possibly controlled drugs. If this option becomes a reality there will be great potential for practice nurses and ANPs to be more responsive to patient needs and provide clients with a faster access to treatment. Eligibility to prescribe will depend upon completion of suitable preparation and from September 2001 this training will become an integral part of the curriculum for specialist practice education programmes, and prescribing competencies will be an essential element of assessment. Upon completion of these updated programmes practitioners will be qualified as nurse prescribers and those who already hold this title can complete a 'stand alone' preparation. The outcome of all this is now awaited and it remains to be seen what will happen to practice nurses.

Table 1.4: Possible extension of prescribing authority

Independent prescribers	Professionals who are responsible for the initial assessment of the patient for devising the broad treatment plan, with authority to prescribe the medicines required as part of that plan, eg. family planning nurses, tissue viability nurses, chiropodists and podiatrists, specialist physiotherapists, optometrists.
Dependent prescribers	Professionals who are authorised to prescribe certain medicines for patients whose condition has been diagnosed or assessed by an independent prescriber within an agreed assessment and treatment plan, eg. specialist diabetes nurses, specialist asthma nurses, specialist palliative care nurses, pharmacists in specialist areas, pharmacists carrying out review of patient's medication.

Practice nursing today

While prescribing remains an important issue, practice nurses continue to develop services and deliver quality care despite political confusion. Nurses remain the first points of contact for many patients offering an efficient and effective health care service. The listening, teaching and support role they provide has become evident, together with recognition of intimate care that supports psychological closeness and sensitivity (Bryan, 1995). The practice nurse role has had an increasing emphasis on health promotional activities, which has resulted in excellent outcomes in helping people change their lifestyles. Practice nurses have proved invaluable in helping people lose weight, encouraging compliance with treatment, providing disease management advice and initiating coping mechanisms for clients. Such nurses have began to take on many innovative roles and the ability to do this in an independent and autonomous fashion has led to recent confusion about when to use the title practice nurse and when to use the title NP. Indeed, there are many role commonalties which overlap and attempts to pinpoint the differences have been made in *Table 1.1*. There are many problems and issues arising around role characteristics and these are discussed in detail in the following chapter.

At its inception from the USA, the NP concept was viewed as an extension of the traditional nursing role, containing elements of medical history-taking, physical examination and medical referral. Fundamental to this role is the philosophy of independent practice, being able to work autonomously and providing direct access for patients.

Because of the similarities with role characteristics between practice nurse and NP, it is impossible to try to offer rigid differences. What is evident is that practice nurses utilise the main characteristics and skills of NPs. Distinction lies in the amount and type of knowledge behind their actions, supported by the level of training and education. The main importance is that, whatever the title, patients understand who they are seeing and that this person is the correct one to meet their needs. If the UKCC have their way, with the introduction of a higher level of practice all titles will be a thing of the past.

Until recently, practice nurses remain in the unique position of being employed by GPs, although there is uncertainty about their future management. The varying employment conditions in terms of incremental pay, sick and maternity leave, educational opportunities, grading and appraisal have left many nurses feeling undervalued, isolated and tempted by the stable and uniform employment conditions of Trusts. Purchasing authorities are always eager to gain management control over practice nurses and this is not always from the incentive of wanting to be helpful to practice nurses. The benefits of this stable employment bring with it the traditional constraints of nursing management and bureaucracy, which is not the solution. Practice nurses now have established positions within general practice and provide a sought-after service by purchasers, GPs and clients, and are in an ideal position to argue their worth. GP employment brings with it a different working relationship, with opportunities to negotiate pay and conditions. As Poole (1999) argues, now is the time for practice nurses to undertake some serious self-evaluation in terms of proving their worth to employers, patients and communities.

In an endeavour to sell themselves, there is no reason why practice nurses should not become self-employed, setting up their own terms and conditions in competing for business. They may even wish to start up provider units or dynamic services to meet the round the clock primary care predicted to be the future by Lilley (1999). The model of general practice primary care with its restricted surgery hours and environment clashes with the ideology of being visible and accessible and in places where people are. For Lilley (1999) future services lie in providing walk-in-centres at railway stations and supermarkets and it would seem practice nurses could have much to offer in satisfying this need.

The potential lies in realising that service provision does not have to be locked within the medical domain, and as Reveley (1998) points out:

Who does what in relation to patient care is becoming increasingly irrelevant in the fast changing world of health care.

Where there is a need for medical input nurses can employ GPs, the reality of this has been tested before in the nurse-led pilot scheme of Catherine Baraniak.

In attempting to become successful in the future, nurses need to believe in what they now have to offer and from what they have learnt in the past. Traditionally, nurses have been indoctrinated to conform and obey the medical profession and this has been enforced through training and years of nursing practice. It is rare for nurses to own their self-worth and value their contributions. The challenge is to overcome the past and embrace the future in developing roles. Advanced practice is the natural next step for practice nurses, the parameters of which are determined essentially by individual imagination and ingenuity. Practice nurses need to continue to function within a role that facilitates individual ideals and independent practice, and incorporate opportunities for taking expertise further. The unique significance of this is assured in the role of the ANP.

2

Defining the meaning of advanced practice

> *I predict that in the year 2000 the nursing spin*
> *doctors will be meeting regularly for deep and*
> *meaningful discussions to decide what to call the*
> *latest super-advanced advanced specialist super-*
> *duper nurse practitioner.*
>
> Wedderburn Tate, 1997

Debates have been, and still are, taking place over what constitutes advanced practice and the term advanced nurse practitioner (ANP). While the concept of advanced practice is not new and has been talked about in Britain for many years, the nature of advanced practice remains unclear and the role itself has yet to be defined. The meaning and interpretation of the ANP role is also subject to world-wide variation.

Advanced nursing practice has been submerged in different role functions which causes confusion, there is a plethora of expanded role titles such as 'advanced practitioner', 'nurse consultant', 'clinical nurse specialist' and 'nurse practitioner' all of which are used synonymously with the concept of progressing practice. Apart from lack of commonality of terms there is also an ambiguity regarding level of preparation for the role, and whether it should be within the remit of line management or embedded entirely in clinical practice. This chapter hopes to explore the history and evolution of the ANP and make sense of the ambiguities in order to offer some operational and conceptual definitions of this rich and dynamic role.

Attempts to set standards for advanced practice were made in by the UKCC (1990), where, 'The standard, kind and content for advanced practice will be specified by the Council'. Despite this initial move and official announcement regarding some form of standardisation of advanced practice, there has been little progress. Today there is still no recordable qualification of advanced practice and no consensus about the nature; scope or criteria for advanced practice.

Historical milestones in advanced nursing practice

In nursing there has been, and still is, a need to define role parameters and to articulate a clear pathway of career structure. The challenge to undertake this was initially taken up by the UKCC in *The Future of Professional Practice* (UKCC, 1994) who proposed three spheres of practice:

- professional
- specialist
- advanced.

Within this definitive document key differences were made in relation to role preparation and definition. This was seen as a concrete commitment by the Council to develop the concept of advanced practice and a clear intention to try to recognise what advanced practice really entailed. This was a substantive beginning in seeing advanced practice as a new and distinct horizon, where it was 'not an additional layer of practice to be superimposed on specialist nursing,' but instead an 'important sphere of professional practice' (UKCC, 1994). The impetus was set together with the potential for creating a form of career ladder for nurses to aspire to.

The Council cascaded further ideas of advanced practice with adjusting the boundaries of future practice, pioneering and developing new roles and enriching professional practice as a whole. There was also clear identification of ANPs as, 'specially prepared nurses who are working in roles which demand a lot of nursing experience, education at Masters degree level, and nursing skills that contribute to meeting the complex needs of vulnerable people and the need to be continuously questioning the fundamentals and boundaries of nursing' (UKCC, 1994). Following this, the UKCC encouraged the development of masters programmes. Universities were hot off the mark to run their own courses on advanced practice. Sanctioning a course and thinking that achievement of it would entitle the individual to become an expert was perhaps also a little naïve

This should have been a major turning point in nursing. The opportunity to establish advanced practice was there, yet the nursing profession failed to take up the challenge and capitalise on the initiative given to it. Despite the success of some universities to create ANPs, the professional world outside has not welcomed them with open arms. This is not surprising as the market was flooded with the creation of other similar roles of varying titles, developed at diploma and degree levels by universities keen to jump on the bandwagon for the market now demanding autonomous practitioners. Such courses have also been guilty of promoting medical models of practice in an attempt to train nurses to fill in the gaps created by the reduction in junior doctor and GP hours, the latter being taken up, at this time, by fund-holding initiatives and paperwork. This momentum was encouraged and supported by government funds to create nurse practitioner type role and courses, all of which left behind the impression that all extended roles implied the medicalisation of nursing. Failure to be prescriptive by the UKCC and to lay down the blueprint for the standards expected of this role, left the door open for the market economy to step in. The destiny of advanced practice is now in the balance and in danger of losing its deserved future. What has been created is frustration, disillusionment and discrepancy, as highlighted by Frost (1998):

> *The debate about 'advanced' nursing practice has become so vexed that those responsible for organising professional courses are discouraged from using the term 'advanced' in course titles, for fear of confusing participants and their funding source.*

The UKCC's failure to set a clinical framework meant that what could have been the potential impetus for clarification of advanced practice, turned out to be nothing more than a gesture. The Council avoided the issues of advanced practice and left nursing and midwifery to decide on the possibilities. The lack of any progression in nursing since 1990, and the failure of its professional body to grasp opportunity, to vocalise worth and show value in expertise is perhaps further proof of nursing's, 'relative academic and professional immaturity and insecurity' (Nolan *et al*, 1998), and a symptom of its tendency for modest approaches lest nurses all try to claim too much and end up looking ridiculous in the process (Robinson, 1994).

There was a need to reach a clear consensus on defining advanced practice, and to take the lead in further developing the collective efforts of the past which valued expert advanced practice:

> *Members of the nursing profession need to hold steadfastly before them a vision of what nursing can become. A continued focus on how the concept of expertise relates to the essence of nursing will help nurses continue to value their artistic abilities.*

Hampton, 1994, p. 23

Historically, advanced practice has been left with false impressions, ignorance and lack of acknowledgement. Little has been achieved to address the nature of advanced practice. ANPs have inherited a legacy of inter-professional struggles and tensions, and it is up to them to create their own recognition and show their unique worth and pioneer practice. However, this role does have some frameworks to follow and advanced practice has become well established in America.

Models of advanced practice

Many writers have attempted to explain advanced practice from various perspectives, yet there is no overall consensus because of the difficulties in trying to define what constitutes levels of performance and expertise. A major assumption of advanced practice is that ANPs are experts who use critical thinking as an added dimension to their expertise and that this not only initiates creativity but also lifts practice into the realms of great depth and vision.

Advanced nursing practice is undoubtedly different from basic level nursing as Styles (1996) characterises it as being:

- specialised in its focus and the population it serves
- expanded in forms of knowledge and skill
- complex regarding aspects of clinical judgement and its challenges and
- independent in terms of autonomous decision-making.

Several theorists have developed models which incorporate this conceptual framework, and the exploration of such models may help to illuminate the nature of advanced practice, for models help to explain, justify and support levels of practice by providing a conceptual representation of reality. Within all models is the notion that ANPs reach the pinnacle of performance in their discipline, becoming experts who 'pursue, capture and master operative knowledge in a specific field or endeavour' (Hampton, 1994, p. 16).

Many of the models within the literature elaborate on or follow the work undertaken by Benner (1984). In her landmark research Benner offered a model of seven domains of expert nursing; within these lie 31 different competencies evident within clinical practice. These domains are:

- the helping role
- administrating and monitoring therapeutic interventions and regimens
- effective management of rapidly changing situations
- the diagnostic and monitoring function
- the teaching-coaching function
- monitoring and ensuring the quality of health care practices
- organisational and work role competencies.

From these domains can be seen the concept of sub-role components of advanced practice in the form of teacher, researcher and evaluator of care. Within this model emphasis is placed on the performance of sophisticated skills and role proficiency, together with specialised front line knowledge. This specialist knowledge is vital to advanced practice and expertise, as it is the essential component of knowing from the broader context, involving a heightened sense of responsibility and possibility (Davies, 1995). Benner's work draws heavily on the concept of expertise and expert nurses, which is relevant to the notion of advanced practice. For Benner (1985):

> *The hallmarks of clinical expertise are an in-depth knowledge of a particular clinical (client or group) population, advanced recognition abilities, and increased use of past whole situations or situation-specific referents for understanding the clinical situation.*

p. 41

ANPs are expert nurses who are highly experienced practitioners capable of excelling. Experiential knowledge is an important feature of advanced practice and inherent within this is an expert performer who no longer relies on analytical principle but has an, 'intuitive grasp of each situation' (Benner, 1984). The picture evolves of ANPs having heightened perceptual awareness and ability to decipher relevant information despite confusing patterns, grasping a situation holistically and rapidly, often below the level of conscious awareness, very much like mastering the skill of riding a bicycle.

Expert practice within Benner's model is reached following an ordinal progression of stages from that of novice to expert, which seems logical, for as Darbyshire indicated (1994, p. 757), 'the person does not move in a lockstep fashion from one level to another'. The end continuum is advanced practice, the ultimate goal to be reached in nursing. It seems inevitable that advanced practice is embodied within the promotion of nursing itself. Individuals pass through stages of skill acquisition to become experts and what stands out is that there is a progression from following abstract rules and detached analytical behaviour to, 'involved skilled behaviour based on an accumulation of concrete experiences and unconscious recognition of new situations as similar to whole remembered ones' (Dreyfus and Dreyfus, 1986, p. 35).

Benner emphasises the use of situations to explain expert practice, which is not always useful in trying to understand the knowledge base or behaviour behind ANPs. As Thompson *et al* (1990) suggest, Benner prefers to look for expertise in the situation, not the individual. For some, the concept of advanced practice is clearly linked to personality and behaviour as well as circumstances.

Fenton (1985) attempted to identify some form of behavioural characteristics, in terms of the skills involved within the clinical judgement expressed by Benner. Fenton introduced the additional domain of the 'consulting role', which focused on the characteristic of influencing others and the behaviour in doing so, such as leadership skills. Leadership is a core competency and characteristic of ANPs, being linked at the same time to vision, risk taking, mentoring and the empowerment of followers (*Chapter 6*).

Calkin (1984) developed a model which also had a different approach to explain advanced practice, this was developed from a perspective which focused on management and aimed at showing nurse administrators how to recognise advanced practice in personnel policies. Instead of focusing the identification of advanced practice on roles, the emphasis lay in proving how ANPs perform under different sets of circumstances, articulate practice and practice needs. Calkin was explicit in identifying advanced practice in terms of clinical judgement and the distinguishing ability to analyse situations and effect change through expertise. This model offers a view of ANPs in respect of their functions and thinking and achieving positive responses to improving the quality of care. The picture therefore emerges of an ANP who is an expert; capable of high levels of clinical practice underpinned by a background of specialist frontline and experiential knowledge. There is also an assumption of certain role characteristics such as that of leader, consultant, change agent, researcher and evaluator of care.

Distinguishing characteristics of advanced practice

From the models outlined, it is evident that none are entirely developed in distinguishing advanced practice or in portraying core values or universal meaning. Darbyshire (1994) claims that, 'It is simply not possible to explicate a complex human experience such as expert nursing in formal, representational propositions which will predict or identify the criteria of expertise' (p. 757).

While emphasis has been made to the role competencies of advanced practice there exists a general view that advanced practice is not a role but a way of thinking and seeing the world based on clinical knowledge, a personal descriptor that can be seen to belong to a person (Salussolia, 1997). This being the case, it seems logical to believe that attributes should follow the person and be transferable into any area of care they choose to practice. Some might argue with this, questioning the transferability of advanced practice, as to become an expert in a field means to stay in this area building up clinical expertise within a specific range and depth of knowledge, it would not seem realistic to achieve this within all clinical areas. Fulbrook (1998) agrees that advanced practice is based in one specific area, and that it is only the core aspects that might be transferable.

Despite the inconsistencies the specific attributes of the ANP cannot be ignored, particularly as the fluid nature and scope of this role inevitably demands certain personality traits of the practitioner. Sutton and Smith (1995) offer significant ideas regarding attributes symbolic of advanced practice, supported by the notion that nursing should rely less on scientific and objective aspects and more on fostering a sense of the individual. An important attribute was thought to be the characteristic of valuing uncertainty, which is perceived as opportunity for growth and development and a chance to legitimise former experience, which has evolved from a well-developed view of the unpredictability of human interaction and a response to illness and health. This coincides with the views of Fulbrook (1998) that advanced practice is about the ability to practice outside the rules. ANPs must also be able to have a clear vision of the future and be seen as achieving high levels of credibility strengthened by their continued self-evaluation and reflection. ANPs, therefore, must have a strong belief in self-worth and an ability to be self-critical.

The attributes of individuals are important in recognising advanced practice and while clinical competence is important, Smith (1995) sees a caring personality as vital to success, with the core of advanced practice lying within nursing's disciplinary perspective on human-environment and caring interrelationships that facilitate health and healing (Smith, 1995).

Emerging themes

Throughout the literature the ANP is associated with many attributes which are as varied as are individual opinions and experiences. It could be considered that advanced practice has two dimensions to it: the scope of practice and the level of performance. The scope of the role encompasses many sub-roles identified in the literature, some of which have been touched on earlier, including the role of researcher, evaluator of care, manager, consultant, educator, role model, change agent, collaborator, leader and mentor (*Table 2.1*).

These roles are not exclusive and it could not be suggested that unless all are utilised the individual is not an ANP. The ANP role will develop individually and in response to demands within the specialism and geographical area; the role will also evolve according to individual strengths, interests, beliefs and limitations. Advanced practice is not about sometimes incorporating these sub-role components, but about implicitly integrating them as a sound foundation, utilising each aspect as the circumstance prescribes.

It may be considered that no one nurse can fulfil such a multifaceted clinical role, yet, it is feasible if it is considered that sub-role components do not have to be of equal importance or significance. The role, however, needs to fulfil the notion of advanced practice by the UKCC (1990) in that, 'advanced practice reflects a range of skills which incorporate direct care, education, research, management, involvement in health policy-making and development of strategies.'

Table 2.1: Operational role competencies of advanced practice	
Researcher, Evaluator of care	Improves the quality of care by utilising scholarly inquiry, nursing theory and application of existing research into daily clinical practice. Supports others to carry out research. Contributes to research and evaluates care.
Change agent	Has confidence and courage to take risks. Able to shape and translate the political environment in which nursing functions. Facilitates clinical change from innovation and extensive experience.
Collaborator	Inspires collaborative vision. Effective communicators and professional networkers.
Leader, Consultant	Pacesetters who shape the future of nursing and client care from vision and clinical expertise.
Role model	A confident, credible practitioner, dynamic and innovative, acting as an example and actually living their ambitions, beliefs and values.
Mentor, Educator	Develops credible methods of expert guidance and education to enable others to gain and retain clinical knowledge. Disseminates new knowledge and information through publications and presentations. A staff, patient and student educator.

The level of performance within advanced practice is linked implicitly to that of an expert which is embodied in experiential, aesthetic, personal, theoretical, scientific and clinical knowledge and judgement that informs practice. The crux to explaining this level is perhaps the main problem when trying to define advanced practice, which is a little like pushing water uphill, as it is easier to see what an ANP does than describe the level of judgement that underpins it. Disclosing and articulating a unique level is complex, what is certain is that it includes a plane that is able to break new ground, challenge vision, push boundaries and reach excellence, and all performed with the client as the centre of that ideal. It is generally felt that advanced practice equates with a Master's level degree although the rationale for this tends to vary. Masters degree level of preparation would seem obvious if the assumption exists that performance should equate with high levels of knowledge, and a role underpinned by commitment to excellence necessitating masterly thought and education.

Within the USA there appears to be a unanimous belief that masters education is a key element to preparation for advanced practice and should remain so (Woods, 1997). There is, however, incongruity within the academic levels between Britain and the States, where an MSc in many instances compares to the level of BSc in Britain a 'ratchet' lower (Paniagua, 1998). The significance of this is important in defining advanced practice, particularly as noted before, Britain tends to follow the lead of America in such issues, and academic institutions need to know the level of attainment for advanced practice and the correct level of competence behind its preparation.

Defining advanced practice in general practice

Practice nurses are in an ideal position to have an affinity with the underpinnings of advanced practice because of the boundary jurisdiction and diversity of their role. This role is one that possesses the opportunity for growth and innovation, essential for advanced practice. The history of practice nursing reveals a role that has overcome many influences and challenges in the past and its survival has shown that as a discipline it can be both flexible and resilient, a useful reputation on which to build an advanced role, where risk is fundamental (see *Chapter 1*). To exercise this role, however, needs a certainty of knowledge and the freedom of autonomy.

Current research supports evidence that the majority of practice nurses are already working autonomously (Cooksley, 1995; Paniagua, 1995), defined by Keenan (1999) as the exercise of considered, independent judgement to effect a desirable outcome. There has been previous argument to suggest that practice nurses are not autonomous as their work is medicalised and prescribed in some aspects by doctors (Smith, 1994). This is confusing autonomy with autocracy. There is a distinction between autocracy, defined by Partridge (1957) as absolute government, and autonomy defined as the right of the institution to govern itself. Practice nurses work with authority to act and make independent decisions offering a service that complements medical practice. Practice nurses have been able to develop their autonomy because there is no clearly defined professional or nursing line management behind them to impose restrictions. This is an advantage as it places nurses in an ideal position to negotiate working relations with doctors, a benefit also for the development of ANP roles, which may require collaborative decision-making.

While practice nurses fulfil roles similar to their GP colleagues they mostly enjoy the freedom to be innovative, providing care that is perceived as more holistic and humanistic. This role incorporates the independent running of clinics, provision of a first point of contact for patients, dealing with initial problems, offering a wealth of practical treatments, health promotion and disease management advice with long term preventive strategies and supervision. The value of such work has provided the opportunity for some to become partners with GPs in decision-making and in care as 'junior partners'. Such role developments are all conducive to substantiating the underpinning autonomy of advanced practice and indicate already the potential to pioneer practice.

Educational responsibilities considered a traditional part of the ANP role are also fundamental to the practice nurse role and there is no shortage of practice nurses who have the potential to be excellent community practice teachers. Practice nurses have been noted to have a key role in the education of pre-registration nursing students (Carter, 1997) providing valuable placement experience, facilitating learning from a wealth of experience and through examples of role modelling. There is an increasing emphasis on health promotional activities provided by practice nurses in which the teaching of patients plays a vital part. Bryan (1995) identified that practice nurses themselves rated teaching patients about health as one of the most important parts of their role.

A further domain relevant to practice nursing is health assessment. This includes the skill of eliciting information and applying the decision-making process once it has been gained. For advanced practice this will include one step further into that of the physical examination. With increasing patient dependency and advances in monitoring technology the nurse is increasingly playing a major role in physical assessment of clients. The development of the practice nurse role into disease management, in areas of women's health, diabetes and asthma has resulted in nurses learning specific skills in order to provide holistic care. To develop advanced practice in the realms of health assessment would mean practice nurses only have to extend their skills.

Many university programmes now include modules or actual courses on physical health assessment for nurses, particularly practice nurses, in response to consumer demand and in recognition of the evolutionary process nursing is undergoing in skill assessment, guided by a nursing knowledge, orientation and emphasis. Synder (1995) believes that ANPs possess a vast store of information that they need to publish in order to share what is successful and identify what needs further study. Effective interpersonal communication is also an important aspect of advanced practice, for which publishing is an easily accessible option. Authorship is beginning to become customary practice for practice nurses, helped no doubt by the many skills already acquired within the role, such as undertaking literature reviews prior to developing protocols, audit or practice profiling. The last few years has witnessed the creation of journals specifically for practice nurses such as *Practice Nursing* and *Practice Nurse*. Practice nurses are influential as editorial board members for these journals, and many practice nurses are actively involved as peer reviewers for the articles submitted.

Practice nursing is receiving increasing media coverage and many formats exist in which to present research and share professional perspectives and networks, such as at regional and national levels in practice nurse conferences. Many practice nurses are increasingly involved in organising or speaking in local study day events, forums or meetings. As a discipline, practice nursing is gradually establishing a body of knowledge and experience which affords visibility and is signalling to others that it is capable of high levels of practice and in improving the quality of patient care. Innovative practice is essential to the ANP role and there is no lack of published examples. Hyde (1997), for example, sees the work of two nurses in Berkshire as particularly imaginative and inventive. These practice nurses analysed their caseload profiles and identified the need to implement an arthritis clinic. There is also undeniable innovation in the pioneering role of Barbara Stillwell, a practice nurse who implemented the nurse practitioner role concept in Britain, and Barbara Burke-Masters who fought relentlessly to provide a doctor surrogate service for vagrant alcoholics.

There are many avenues open for practice nurses to be at the cutting edge of health care and to move into innovative practice arenas. The White Paper, *The new NHS – modern, dependable* (DoH, 1997) was a firm endorsement of the potential within primary care and the development of primary care groups (PCGs) and primary care trusts (PCTs) will be the forum in which nurses can exert influence. Practice nurses need to be involved or strongly vocal at all structural levels of the PCGs. Those practice nurses already involved as PCG board members will have a direct influence on budget decisions for community provision and the power to lead on issues of quality care, public health and professional development. The opportunity is there for practice nurses to use their skills and knowledge to shape a brand new community health service for the new Millenium.

In summary, practice nurses are often working in technically advanced, autonomous and clinically demanding arenas of practice with opportunities to lead nursing and take on board the multifaceted role of advanced practice. However, these nurses by virtue of their position are not ANPs, this remains a distinct sphere of nursing that is ever evolving and equates with mastery and experiential knowledge gained over time, with academic credibility and with skills built from a wealth of clinical experience and vision. The role of the practice nurses can provide the framework and transferable core in which to develop advanced practice, and those that choose to do so are in an optimal position. The range of possibility to develop advanced practice is infinite within general practice, and it will depend on the aspirations, desires and motivation of individuals to carry it through. Practice nurses could find that they have a unique background of knowledge and experience in which to demonstrate to many what advanced practice can really be about.

The future of advanced practice

The future of advanced practice is unclear, as the ambiguity in Britain regarding the ANP role has led to a paradigm shift within the UKCC towards supporting a higher level of practice rather than setting standards for advanced practice as, '... A checklist of standards would be in direct conflict with the dynamic and autonomous nature of advancing practice' (UKCC, 1997). The UKCC now seem set to examine the practice characteristics of practitioners working in clinical practice and the outcomes against which this can be assessed are based on a level, 'significantly higher than initial registration' (UKCC, 1999). The UKCC are also examining the possibility of higher level practitioners holding a mandatory mark against their name on the register and the need to regularly notify intention to practice. Little is known as to whether there will be recognition of the master's level prepared ANP role, or whether the introduction of new standards will just muddy the waters further. As Frost (1998) points out, 'if you're in a hole don't keep digging.' The draft standard does seem to mention characteristics already attributable to advanced practice, with comments that higher level practitioners should lead practice, work across professional and organisational boundaries, develop others and introduce innovation and change. In identifying 'how' practitioners work at a higher level of practice as well as 'what' they do raises a dilemma in that the UKCC is not acknowledging any 'why'. The acting on this is the essence of advanced practice. There is also confusion about interpretations of the term level of practice, for the UKCC this seems to be the identification of uniform distinction, not a reference to level in terms of bringing up or down, for which advanced practice slips into the top plane, being, in principle, the higher level of practice.

It is to be hoped that the concepts of advanced practice already identified will not be lost in any quest to get rid of titles or any good established university programmes diffused in an attempt to accommodate new ideas. Whatever the future, the ANP role will continue to be provocative and there will be years of unpredicted change and uncertainty ahead. It would seem sensible to suggest that instead of following in the footsteps of others, those wishing to advance practice should set off ahead and leave a path behind for others to follow.

3
The nature of advanced practice consultations

The round faced man in black entered, and
dissipated all doubts on the subject by beginning
to talk.
My First Acquaintance with Poets, William Hazlitt

The consultation is a powerful process which holds many agendas, controls and consequences. For practice nurses this is an effective tool in which to persuade, advise, manipulate and instruct patients. For patients however, the consultation is the only way of interacting with a health professional and the first opportunity to express worries and fears that need answers that may change their lives. In advanced practice the consultation provides the opportunity for the advanced nurse practitioner (ANP) to meet the expectations of patients and provide the expert professional judgement central to its overall competence and recognition.

The consultative role in general practice is a significant aspect of practice nursing and provides quality, depth and comprehensiveness to most encounters, yet the culture of nursing has not recognised the consultation process as an important strategy when providing patient care. Most of the literature surrounding consultation focuses on medical interactions and interviews, acknowledging it as the cornerstone of medical practice (Thompson, 1988).

A substantial amount of practice nurse time is spent in consultations and it is therefore important to consider this unique interaction and the clinical expertise involved in a different occupational arena. The dynamics of consultations hold the key to discovering the artistry of practice nursing as well as being a vital initiative for delivering the reality of creative, quality care which is expected of advanced practice.

Defining consultations

Caplan (1970) sees the consultation as a process of communication between the health professional and client, which can be systematically taught, applied and analysed. This encounter, however, is complex and consists of evolving events, each phase having its own behaviours, procedures and consequences. Most patients initiate consultations to:

- meet an identified need
- find relief from discomfort
- recover well being or a loss of function
- gain verification of illness
- receive advice.

For nurses the purpose of the encounter is different and may be to reach an accurate diagnosis, provide appropriate answers or goals, initiate treatment and manage time effectively in order to meet the needs of the next patient. The encounter is distinct from many other interactions as both parties try, from their different agendas, to reach a common goal. Also, unlike many other interactions, this meeting takes place at a specific place within restricted time limits and conditions, has a pattern of formal events and there is inevitably some degree of competence gap between the participants. For most patients the consultation remains the most common means of interacting within general practice, an avenue in which they have events to relate, fears to alleviate, occasions for favours, desires for information and the need to confirm lay beliefs. Neighbour (1987) views the consultation as an actual journey as the patient expects things to change from one state of affairs to another, as a result of being seen.

Models of consultation

There are many different models of consultations, eg. the doctor/ patient consultation model and the process consultation model (Schein, 1969) (*Table 3.1*). It is useful to be aware of these not only to understand practice, but also to think of relevant strategies to deal constructively with patients.

Table 3.1: Consultation models (Shein, 1969)		
Source	Patient characteristics	Nurse characteristics
The doctor-patient consultation model	Seeks professional advice and complies.	Defines the problem and offers a solution.
The process consultation model	Seeks professional advice in a partnership with professional. Patient accepts the solution and internalises the methods for the future.	Works in partnership with patient in a patient-defined context.

The doctor-patient model is probably the most common and constitutes the medical approach of diagnosing the problem and prescribing the solution. This model offers transferability to nursing consultations and is useful when there is limited time or the problem is straightforward. The idea of adopting a medical approach to care is not always popular with some nurses as it may be thought to conflict with the ideals of nursing, although in reality, it can enhance them. Medical and nursing care will always be different and there will always be role overlap particularly in expanding nursing roles, although this does not mean that approaches will be the same.The spirit of nursing should always be the philosophy of holism and the concentration of the effects of illness rather than the disease itself. Consultations using the medical framework will be different because of the aspirations of nurses towards a patient-centred approach rather than the disease-centred focus of medicine. As highlighted by Fawcett (1984) nursing focuses on the person requiring care, on their environment and at the time of contact the nature of the health to illness continuum. The use of this model, however, tends to be based on the assumptions about the patient such as compliance, good communication ability and willingness to accept the solution given.

The other model of Edgar Schein (1969) seen in *Table 3.1*, the process consultation model, focuses more on working collaboratively with patients to assess the problem and the help needed to solve it. This is probably more in tune with nursing as it assumes working in partnership with patients to provide the solutions. Consultation using this framework can be pro-active, directed towards anticipating future problems and thinking of ways to prevent them, and reactive, which is directed towards solving the problem itself. Techniques can be applied within this model as suggested by Blake and Moulton (1983), and these have been highlighted in *Table 3.2*.

Table 3.2: Consultative interventions (Blake and Moulton, 1983)

Intervention	Example		Consultation actions
Acceptance	ANP encourages the sharing of feelings, such as the powerlessness felt through inability to change a marital problem.	1	Listen in order to fully understand feelings.
		2	Do not agree or disagree — instead try to encourage the patient to talk and realise their feelings.
		3	Refrain from being judgmental and help the patient to find a solution.
Catalytic	ANP tells the patient of the importance of elevating the foot during the day to improve a venous ulcer, which is not healing.	1	Avoid outright suggestions. Instead, provide support and encouragement in order for the patient to make the decisions.
		2	Try to be non-authoritarian and provide logical, constructive information relevant to the patient.
		3	Ask the patient to explain their problems and use this as a basis for resolution.
Confrontation	ANP presents the fact that unless the patient stops smoking, they cannot continue taking the combined oral contraceptive pill.	1	Do not personally attack the client's views or values.
		2	Challenge the client's action logically, probing for the motives and causes of the present situation.
		3	Offer your own thoughts on the problem, presenting data to add support.
Prescriptive	ANP explains that it is advisable not to wear nylon underwear and trousers each day, in order to prevent vaginal thrush.	1	By acting authoritatively, tell the patient the logical solution.
		2	Offer praise and encouragement where possible and try to understand the patient's situation.
Theory principles	ANP teaches examination of the testes to a patient by applying behaviour theory.	1	Offer support and understanding and do not be judgmental.
		2	Provide strategies and introduce theories for problem-solving.
		3	Use techniques to help the patient internalise the concepts.

The practice nurse's choice of which intervention is appropriate will depend upon the patient and the problem, and consultation may involve using one or more together. The techniques are:

* **Acceptant intervention**, which can be used to help the patient clarify emotional reactions to objectively understand and deal with problems.

* **Catalytic intervention**, which is a way of providing patients with information in order to clarify understanding and raise awareness.

* **Confrontation intervention**, which is used to provide the patient with the realisation of their individual value systems and beliefs in an indisputable way, allowing them to consider alternative values in order to redirect behaviour.

* **Prescriptive intervention**, which requires the nurse to be more instructive and involves telling the patient outright how to solve the problem.

* **Theory-principle intervention**, which is used as a means of enabling the patient to learn theories, such as behavioural theory, and apply them to problem-solving.

Use of the process/consultation model assumes that patients want to improve situations and be involved in decision-making, and that goals are more effective if applied within the patients' understanding of their strengths and limitations.

Consultation process

The underpinning notion to these models is the process of helping the patient perceive, understand and act upon situations, which is important if the consultative process is to be effective. Consultations used in this way are similar to processes of experiential learning, as nurses need to help patients find and learn different and new methods of behaving in order to overcome problems. This is also closely linked to notions of empowerment, which is seen as a process of transferring power to patients and at the same time creating their positive self-esteem. A core mechanism of the consultation is to promote an alliance with patients that creates a belief in themselves and their ability to handle situations effectively from their strengths, abilities and personal power. Part of this process needs a commitment by the nurse to self and others to become closer to patients in order to understand problems from the patient's perspective and convey this understanding back to them. There is a sense of authentic presence for this interaction where empowerment originates in self-esteem developed through love, interest, genuineness and opportunities for choice. The facilitation of this environment is perhaps affiliated to the perception of Heron (1990) in which practitioners work by the grace within the human spirit, which is believed to be the primary source of effective human behaviour. This helping grace and attunement to experiential reality requires a sense of caring concern for patients as people, an ability which has been seen as one of the most important resources nurses bring to patient care. In fact, this positive concern has been theorised as the defining characteristic of nursing itself (Benner and Wrubel, 1989). Concern with personal interest for others and belief in their worth, dignity and 'irreplaceability' is essential to enhancing nursing care. Patients, who perceive nurses to be caring, experience less distress in the form of depression, anger and anxiety than when they perceive nurses to be lacking in empathy (Olson, 1995). ANPs will be skilful in establishing collaborative relationships with patients and use this to enhance the therapeutic nature and quality of the consultation.

Within the context of general practice, such caring relationships have been identified as essential to consultations and any actions within them (Paniagua, 1997). Practice nurses describe this positive connection with patients as forming a friendship, which, in turn, creates the right environment where patients can feel relaxed and valued. The cultivation of this type of relationship with patients is crucial for effective communication and the creation of a safe environment in which patients can feel secure enough to say what they feel. It is important for patients to have their say, however hesitant, and creating the right ambience is the most important contribution a health professional can give to a consultation. Patients are reluctant to ask questions during consultations, often through fear of being seen as incompetent, from feelings of intimidation and inadequacy. Forming friendships with patients is an essential element of patient interaction, which acknowledges a shared humanity that can overcome obstacles and provide an approach those patients will value and respond to. It is important that patients feel that they are valued during the consultation, and that they are being heard, understood and acknowledged.

In addition to the experience of individualising patient care through friendship, practice nurses have identified the importance of 'knowing' patients (Paniagua, 1997). Specific factors were related to knowing patients, including the experience of caring for patients in general, understanding patients from a knowledge of their actual home environment (perhaps from home visits), from a knowledge of their family backgrounds (as relatives would often inevitably frequent the surgery), and daily lives which were effected when they visited the surgery. Knowing the patient resulted in more positive outcomes, as nurses were able to make more accurate, individual and responsive decisions during consultations based on a larger picture and generic knowledge of patients.

Knowing the patient has also been associated as a characteristic of expert nurses' decision-making relevant to advanced practice. Tanner *et al* (1993) claims that understanding what the patient needs is what makes them expert. Expert-nursing judgement is recognised through a progressive refinement of the ability to gain patient knowledge and devise and select individualised interventions within it. Successful relationships fostered through holistic interaction and a sense of closeness between patient and nurse is the key to effective consultation.

Phases of consultation

To understand the nature of the consultation involves appreciation of the interconnection and relatedness of systems and contexts within it. Consultations are made up of a series of steps and principles. Barron (1989) proposes that with experts the process of events can occur so rapidly that they may not be consciously aware of using them. The stages take place within the format of an interview, described as a purposeful conversation and process of communication in which two or more persons interact to achieve a goal (Croft, 1980). In trying to understand what is happening during the consultation process Neighbour (1987) uses the analogy of the interviewer as using two heads. The second head, the responder, is the intuitive, spontaneous part of the self that forms an internal dialogue that resounds to what takes place, while the real head, the organiser is the one that talks out loud. This image gives the impression of two consultations going on at the same time, the outer loud one between the interviewer and the patient, which could be video recorded and the inner consultation which goes back and forth searching inwards to the memory and the imagination, saying what to do and ask next. If the comments from the second head become too predominant then the interviewer is distracted from the interview. Successful outer consultation with the patient requires having an inner consultation that is effective.

In general, consultation interviews are divided into three stages: opening, operational and finishing (*Table 3.3*) and these steps vary in length and form, and success or problems in any stage can affect the outcome of the others.

The opening stage is the ice breaking that begins the interview and leads into consideration of the request or concern which brought the patient. On initial contact with patients practice nurses use small talk, this may be dismissed as just chatting yet it is an important function as it can be a means of overcoming the initial barriers experienced with interpersonal encounters. This procedure is also better explained in the context of a greeting ritual, where talking on neutral and impersonal grounds reduces threat and allows participants to adjust to each other. This period is important as it forms the basis for the rapport and trust necessary to achieve goals.

During the operational stage, nurse and patient move towards the aim of the interview, which is to determine why the patient is there, whether from a simple need or request, or from a complex problem resulting from a lack of knowledge, capability, confidence or objectivity. Patients' problems are not usually isolated but have physical, psychological and social aspects, which need to be recognised and considered within the whole framework of events. For ANPs this is integral to their expertise, and to understand and assess patients within this context represents an aspect of advanced practice that is holistic and necessary for any pursuit of quality care. Expert care from the understanding of the whole patient, including the physical, spiritual, emotional and cultural needs is an ideal opportunity to demonstrate excellence in nursing care and to promote it professionally as a valued science and art.

Patient problems also need to be understood within the context of their divergent viewpoints; perspectives need to be gained from many aspects such as inaccurate information as well as accurate, general beliefs, previous experience, irrational ideas, fears and misconceptions. People can be selective both about what they want to reveal and the order in which they want to divulge it, this may also be linked to what they define and interpret as relevant or important. In order to implement a holistic approach delivered both competently and humanistically nurses need to use skills during the consultation to assess the whole patient. Such skills are integral to personal qualities and an expertise embedded in the nurse-patient relationship that constitutes excellence in nursing care.

Effective communication is central to interpersonal relations and the ability to facilitate this during this working phase is vital if

Table 3.3: The consultation interview

Interviewing stage	Goal	Strategies	
		Verbal	Non-verbal
Opening	To set the scene in order to establish a relationship within an atmosphere of security, trust and understanding.	To break the ice through chatting and greeting rituals.	Smiling and using eye contact. Appearing friendly and open.
Operational	To gather information in order to establish why the patient has come, and what they want, need and expect. To establish empathy and help the patient understand their strengths, limitations and values. Take action in response to effective communication and determine goals, including patients within the decision-making process. To be able to reach a diagnosis if relevant and provide the correct answers, treatment and support.	Interpret information by funnelling questions. Avoid using leading questions. Responses should be non-judgmental, use tact as the problem is identified and discussed. Use strategies to ensure understanding, eg. asking the patient to repeat what you have said in their own words.	Sit or stand next to the patient, not face to face across the table. Observe the patient's verbal and non-verbal behaviour. Listen to what the patient is not saying as well as actually speaking. Use visual aids, leaflets and diagrams to support explanations.
Finishing	To end the consultation leaving the patient satisfied with the encounter and having clear expectations for the future.	Use clues to indicate the interview has ended, eg. asking the patient to come back in the week.	Make a move to get up and show the patient out.

consultations are to be productive. There needs to be a shared understanding between the nurse and patient if co-operative and co-ordinated behaviour is to take place. Communication however, is seldom what it appears to be, and the critical interior of communication lies in understanding not what is visible but what is invisible and hidden (Reilly and Di Angelo, 1990). The communication process is a challenge during consultation and nurses need to be aware of this.

The starting point for effective communication is through listening to patients and demonstrating that this is happening; paying attention also means attempting to understand the non-verbal signals being emitted. Lack of attention can make the patient feel worthless and ignored, which may restrict disclosure of information as well as limit any discussion. Brill (1973) estimated that in an average consultation one third of the information is given by verbal means and two thirds by non-verbal. Argyle (1978) suggests that the form of non-verbal communication is five times more powerful than the verbal aspect of the message. Nurses need to be receptive to these cues and listening and attending are the two most important elements of therapeutic communication.

There are some useful ground rules within non-verbal communication, which can be incorporated effectively into the operational phase of consultation:

1. Sit or stand next to, not opposite, patients. Spatial behaviour is determined by culture and feelings and can lead to substantial misinterpretation. A desk between professional and patient may be regarded as confrontational and imply a professional power that could inhibit conversation.
2. Adopt an open posture. Ekman and Freison (1972) claim gesture will substitute speech, and body language is more important than words in establishing trust.
3. Lean slightly forward. Using this position as well as an occasional nod of the head has been associated by patients with a higher satisfaction of consultations, and also with regarding practitioners as being warmer, with a more attractive personality (Larsen and Smith, 1981).
4. Maintain eye contact, as facial expression is a powerful transmitter of negative and positive signals and if it is not used it may be perceived by patients as a lack of interest, trustworthiness or attention (Altschul, 1972).

A key element in attempting to improve communication during this part of the consultation is the use of humour. This is often a useful strategy in patient-centred holistic nursing care, and it is thought that nurses who dispense humour will easily establish a rapport with patients. Humour is also effective for the smooth running of interactions and if used in good faith, in the patients interests and in a caring manner, it can be a shortcut to closeness, supportiveness and ultimately a therapeutic mechanism in maintaining or improving well being. The ability to use humour depends on accurate recognition of other people's inner feelings and emotional states by picking up cues from the consultation. Dunn (1993) believes that this is related to synchronicity and being on the same wavelength as patients, which accords with the skills of experts, who see and use patterns in the context of advanced practice.

The nature of relationships during consultation needs insight and a knowledge base which stems from an understanding of human responses. The emphasis on establishing communication and creating the right environment is vital to the main aim of gaining information in order to generate an initial hypothesis, diagnosis or reason for the patients' problems. Problem-solving is not undertaken by the practitioner alone as Croft (1980) identifies, the decision, although strived at through interaction by both partakers in the process, should be predominantly that of the patient. There is a danger that in providing solutions nurses may work from other agendas where professional training inoculates them from patients' real needs and makes them prey to the rhetoric of thinking and believing that they know best (McCormack, 1993).

A great deal of information needs to be obtained from the patient during this operational stage, and skill is needed in deciding what questions to ask and how to ask them. In order to pursue ideas questions should guide the conversation from the general to the more specific which Kahn and Connell (1957) describe as funnelling. In this way the conversation starts with broad, opening questions, which generate more precise and focused questions. In advanced practice experts are able to spread their search of questions quickly, selecting from a wide knowledge base of possibilities, activating a complex system of relationships between cues and questions.

Having acquired all the information a choice has to be made about how to respond to a patient, either by an action such as physical examination with or without treatment, or the giving of advice, or through the setting of future goals. The action should be chosen by involving patients in the decision-making process as Brown *et al* (1992) emphasised one of the common problems felt by patients is that they are uninformed, uninvolved and disassociated from the major part of what is happening to them. Patients are also more likely to comply with an action if they have been involved in choosing it. Once goals have been established and actions undertaken the next stage in the interview is formal closure of the consultation. This involves giving the patient a sense that time is coming to an end. This, like all other phases, relies on effective communication as it should be done smoothly so that the patient does not feel cut off abruptly and that they are left with a sense of achievement and satisfaction. The first stage to closing is often initiated when one participant demonstrates through some verbal or non-verbal clues that the subject has run dry.

The HANDS checkpoint system could be a useful tool to remember and implement as goals to achieve at each consultation. This model needs to be linked to the finger and thumb of the left hand to become an aide memoir and each sub-goal needs to be achieved (*Table 3.4*).

Given the complexity of communication and the interpersonal relationship involved ANPs can play a vital role in developing innovative approaches to patient interactions, in order to enhance and extend quality of nursing care. There is evidence to show that practice nurses already have a long tradition of established patterns of skilful consultation (Paniagua, 1997 seen in *Figure 3.1*) and this can be built upon as part of the dynamic process.

Consultations have the potential to influence patient care and provide a mastery to care that can meet the increasingly challenging and diverse needs of patients. The power of consultations to inform and advance practice makes this an integral aspect of the ANP role and one that can highlight the unique expertise of practice nursing.

Table 3.4: HANDS checkpoint system

Thumb	**H**istory	At the beginning of the consultation during the history-taking, relate thoughts back to the patient to test for accuracy. This prevents misunderstanding and facilitates precision in questioning.
Index finger	**A**ssessment	Following acquisition of information, the patient's needs and problems have to be assessed and goals set. Assessment may involve the art of physical examination to reach a more holistic perspective.
Middle finger	**N**on-verbal communication	This is a reminder to include the patient's non-verbal communication in forming an assessment. Focus also on personal non-verbal communication as this can reinforce expressed interest, help to motivate patients and establish the rapport necessary to achieve communication.
Ring finger	**D**ecision-making and **d**iagnosis	This is the next step and refers to the need to decide upon an action, solution or diagnosis. Make sure that any treatment or management decisions have been made together with the patient. Patients are more likely to comply with any action if they have been involved with choosing it. Decisions should be made within a framework of personal confidence where all actions can be totally justified and undertaken in the patient's best interests.
Little finger	**S**atisfaction and **s**hut down	This involves closing the consultation in a way that leaves the patient feeling a sense of satisfaction rather than feeling hurried away. Proper closure is important as sense of achievement and expectation for the future will also be influenced by it. Personal satisfaction should also be felt that every-thing was remembered, agendas achieved and contingency plans made to pre-empt any unforeseen possibilities.

Figure 3.1: Established patterns of consultation

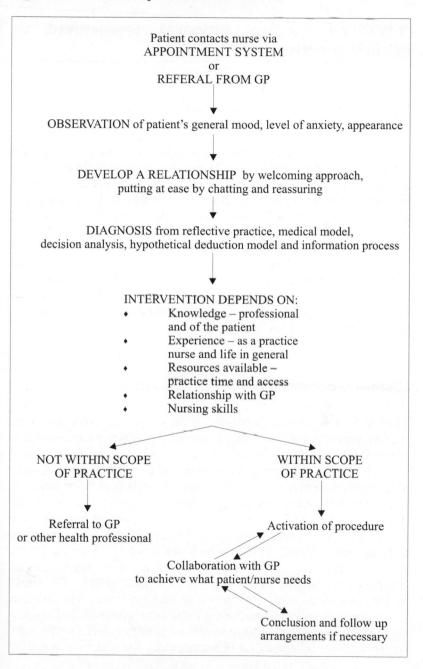

Patient contacts nurse via
APPOINTMENT SYSTEM
or
REFERAL FROM GP

OBSERVATION of patient's general mood, level of anxiety, appearance

DEVELOP A RELATIONSHIP by welcoming approach,
putting at ease by chatting and reassuring

DIAGNOSIS from reflective practice, medical model,
decision analysis, hypothetical deduction model and information process

INTERVENTION DEPENDS ON:
- Knowledge – professional and of the patient
- Experience – as a practice nurse and life in general
- Resources available – practice time and access
- Relationship with GP
- Nursing skills

NOT WITHIN SCOPE
OF PRACTICE

WITHIN SCOPE
OF PRACTICE

Referral to GP
or other health professional

Activation of procedure

Collaboration with GP
to achieve what patient/nurse needs

Conclusion and follow up
arrangements if necessary

4

Advanced nursing physical assessment in general practice

Without prognosis, diagnosis is Godnosis.

Anon

The central aim of practice nurse interaction with patients is to find out the root of their problems in order to help them to do something about them. Physical examination can often be the crux to finding out this information and the ability to do this well increases the potential to offer accurate answers, based on a more holistic and reliable perspective. For many practice nurses, physical examination has already become a natural progression of their role, in congruence with their work as either nurse practitioner, overseers of clinics or as first line contacts for patients. The role of undertaking physical examination also underpins that of the advanced nurse practitioner (ANP), which highlights the easy sub-role transferability from practice nursing into advanced practice.

Historical background to role expansion

There are many debates at present, about expanding roles into what is often perceived as traditionally medical practice. Fears exist that undertaking techno-medical activities erodes into the fundamental heart of nursing as a caring profession and that nurses are in danger of losing their core nursing skills in the rush to become mini-doctors. The source of these misgivings probably stems from the initial driving force behind nursing role expansion, which has been the change in junior doctor working. The major influence has been the Calman report (DoH, 1993a) which set out to standardise junior doctor education, revoking tasks that are repetitive, routine and of 'no clear educational value' and the *New Deal* (NHS ME, 1991) initiatives underpinning a reduction in doctors' hours. The solution to any foreseen problems stemming from these incentives had already been calculated by the Department of Health (DoH, 1990) who suggested that tasks considered unnecessary for education could be undertaken by others such as, 'appropriately trained nurses'.

It is not surprising that nurses resent becoming vehicles for offloaded medical time or take exception to the view that they should automatically take over the mundane duties of doctors. The issues surrounding physical examination touch on obvious sensitivity and professional boundaries, yet the time is fast approaching for nurses to become mindful of the opportunities within this and to become pro-active instead of reactive in their responses. A persuasive argument exists in considering examination in the light of total care delivery and not as an isolated technical activity, recognising that it is possible to balance caring with technical skills to provide a significantly enhanced service to patients.

As Riev (1994) points out, it is the patient who should take priority in these matters, and it is whether the patient gets a better deal in terms of quality of care or not. While the task of examination may be the same for nurses and doctors, the perspective behind the action will be different with nurses emphasising a more patient-centred assessment (*Table 4.1*).

Table 4.1: Differences in doctors and nurses orientation

Doctors	Nurses
Focuses on symptoms or parts of the patient.	Views the patient as a whole.
Concentrates on what is wrong.	Focuses on what is right as well as wrong.
Assesses from a problem-orientated approach.	Assesses from patient's expressed and felt needs, although problems will be considered.
Reductionist perspective.	Holistic perspective.
Doctor-focused.	Patient-focused.
Disease-centred orientation.	Orientated from a perspective of health promotion, education and primary prevention.
Doctor defines the problem and decides the solution.	Patient and nurse search for the problem and decide on the solution together.
Based on established ideas of universal medical practices and patient rights.	Based on nursing knowledge and experience of past interactions.
Background knowledge is scientific.	Background knowledge based on both science and lived experience.

Any new role will have implications for accountability, and nurses undertaking physical examination skills must be accountable for their actions. The launch of *The Scope of Professional Practice* (UKCC, 1992a) has led the way to encouraging the development of independent practice, as long as practice is underpinned by appropriate education and experience. The Scope document is based on the premise that nurses use their own discretion in extending their role, dictated by the extent to which they acknowledge their individual limitations to practice. The urge to be self-reliant in developing practice is further reinforced by the *Code of Professional Conduct* (UKCC, 1992b) which acts as a yardstick to direct practice. While nurses maintain this code there is no limitation or constraints on practice other than that covered by law, and as Reveley and Money (1998) advise, as long as patients realise that they are seeing a nurse not a doctor.

Nurses wishing to enhance their practice and utilise new skills which inevitably increases their accountability should be aware not only of their obligations to the UKCC but also in law. The purpose of highlighting this is not to frighten nurses or deter them from ever taking on board new skills or increasing their autonomy. It may be helpful to consider that all practitioners have to practice at some time as well as do things for the first time, so the law does not actively seek to prohibit innovation or progression. It is important to be aware of the legal background to specific situations in order to understand the issues and justify and explain decisions.

General principles of professional liability and accountability

The law or 'tort' of negligence is probably the most important civil law nurses need to come to terms with. This branch is concerned with compensation for injuries caused by another's negligence. Negligence is not always an easy case to win as the client has to prove four things:

- that a duty of care existed
- that there was a breach of that duty
- that foreseeable harm was caused
- that harm was a result of that breach of duty (a causal link).

Duty of care

Most would agree that a health professional has a duty of care for the client, this is implicit in the very nature of the patient/nurse relationship which exists upon the basis of caring. A duty of care is not owned universally so this is not always so clear cut. Difficulties may also arise in the case of nurses if the person was not actually a patient or on the nurse's caseload. Duty of care involves situations where there is a pre-existing relationship between parties, where the person giving the advice or undertaking an action holds themselves in the position of having the necessary knowledge and skill, and finally if that person knew or should have known that the other person intended to reply to it.

It is up to the plaintiff to show that duty of care is owed and this is achieved by applying the test case of *Donaghue v Stephenson* [1932]. The principles of this were established following the distress caused by a woman drinking a bottle of ginger beer containing a decomposed snail. The manufactures were seen to have a duty of care by the courts. It was held that, 'A duty existed if a person would be so closely and directly affected by ones acts that one ought reasonably to have them in contemplation as being so affected when directing one's mind to the acts or omissions which are called into question'. This is particularly significant for nurses as it highlights that nurses can be sued not only for what they actually do but also for what they actively do not do. This case subsequently also gave rise to the 'neighbour principle' as the Judge held that reasonable care should be taken to avoid acts or omissions which could be reasonably foreseen as to cause injury to a neighbour.

Breach of duty

In order to establish that a breach of duty has occurred, it is first necessary to establish the standard of care expected. The 'Bolam test' is used to determine the professional standard in similar cases. This case law came from a case *Bolam v Friern Hospital Management Committee* [1957] which dealt with the negligence of a doctor who fractured a patient's skull while administering electro-convulsive therapy. The Judge ruled that a doctor would not be thought negligent if he acted in accordance with the practice or standard accepted by a responsible body of medical men skilled in that particular art. The law, therefore, imposes the duty of care but that the standard is a matter of professional judgement. This test, while relating specifically to doctors, is still applicable to nurses and the standard of that ordinary skilled nurse exercising and professing to have that skill. The problem exists in determining what is the standard of skill for nurses undertaking physical examination; a skill mainly attributed to doctors. As yet there has not been a test case where harm has been caused from examination negligence, so as always this would depend on decisions involving the particular circumstances.

Foreseeable harm and causal link

Following the establishment of a breach of duty it has to be shown that harm should have been reasonably foreseen and avoided. Such a link is not inevitably straightforward, for example in the case of *Barnett v Chelsea and Kensington Hospital Committee* (1969). Here a doctor refused to see a man in casualty who had drunk a cup of tea and was suffering gastro-intestinal problems. The man died and it was subsequently found that the tea had contained arsenic. The widow lost the case as while the doctor could be considered in breach of duty by not seeing the patient, had he have done so he could not have prevented his death. His omission therefore had also not caused the patient's death.

Generally, if nurses practise following the guidelines of the UKCC, protocols and terms of employment in a case of negligence compensation are usually sought from the employers under their vicarious liability to employees. However, this is in no way a safety net for nurses as vicarious liability is dependent on whether the act or omission was within the terms of employment or if nurses went off on a 'frolic' of their own. Nurses can also be sued alongside their employers or by their employers so nurses, particularly ANPs, are advised to seek personal insurance and security against such actions by a body that is particularly sympathetic to the skills and needs of advanced practice, such as the Medical Defence Union and the Royal College of Nursing.

Despite obvious concerns nurses should remember that in any dispute there are several defences available (Dimond, 1997). These include:

- dispute over the facts (cases fail when the defendant denies the facts and the plaintiff cannot show under the balance of probabilities that they are right)
- one of the elements of negligence is missing

- contributory negligence (where the client is partly to blame)
- willing assumption of risk (the person willingly undertook the risk)
- limitation of time (cases have to be commenced within three years of the event).

A thorough knowledge of the law and its implications for practice should pave the way for nurses to provide a more realistic and effective service for patients. This does however mean receiving clinical training. Practice nurses are in an ideal position to acquire coaching as Marsh and Dawes (1995) highlight, experienced GPs are ideal for teaching nurses about diagnosis, and doctors provide expertise in helping practitioners develop history-taking, examination and therapeutic skills (O'Hara Deveraux, 1991). Individual practices can successfully train practice nurse 'in house', and many universities have now devised courses to provide skills in examination and diagnosis, some of which are incorporated within BSc programmes.

Physical assessment skills

Practice nurses have easy access to training to do physical examinations, which have a logical part to play in their role. For ANPs the art of examination is part of the dynamic process in responding to patients' needs and, combined with their expert critical thinking ability, is the key to offering a unique service. Physical examination includes the use of various techniques, the core of which are inspection, palpation, auscultation and percussion. It is useful to understand the basic principles of these procedures as they form part of most systematic examinations and nursing procedures. It is not within the remit of this chapter to explain examination as it relates to each specific part of the body, but rather to provide an overview of the basic techniques. Procedures considered pertinent to the practice nurse role will be covered in more depth.

Inspection

Inspection is the use of visual skills to gather information on anatomy, specifying characteristics such as shape, position, symmetry, size, colour, location and movement, and the patient as a whole. Observation begins as the patient enters the room and continues throughout taking the history and the examination. Pease (1985) points out the importance of identifying non-verbal messages in clothes, personal hygiene and general appearance. It is necessary to be aware of the patient's verbal statements and body language throughout the appointment. Active looking does not include special manoeuvres or instruments but as King (1983) recognises palpation, percussion or auscultation will rarely uncover an abnormality that will not be exhibited in some sign found on inspection. Adeptness in widening and narrowing the perceptual field selectively will come with time and experience. There are a number of suggestions that can help to develop observation skills, including:

1. Think of yourself as a film director and register all you can see on that particular scene without ignoring anything. Silently describe the details of what you are seeing.
2. Tell yourself in your mind what you see.
3. Ask yourself if the patient's body language confirms or disputes what you think.
4. Think whether you are being objective and critical or prejudiced.
5. Listen to what the patient is not telling you as well as what he is telling you.
6. Ask yourself if your observations could be due to possible cultural differences or expectations on your part.
7. Look for clues to confirm what you see and hear, eg. if the patient complains of having very heavy periods, look to see if there is any paleness of the skin. Include use of all senses eg. the smell of smoke on clothing for patients complaining of a productive cough.
8. Write down any specific points and observations as you make them.
9. Be aware of all senses. It is a good reason to shake hands on first meeting as you can detect nervousness perhaps from sweating palms.

Using an auriscope

Inspection is generally restricted to looking with the unaided eye but in a broader sense can include using instruments such as the auriscope. The auriscope provides a source of light and magnification for examining the external auditory canal and tympanic membrane of the ear. There are many instances when practice nurses are required to examine the ear, but probably the most common is for the procedure of ear syringing. Sharp *et al* (1990) claims that 81% of GPs delegate ear syringing routinely to practice nurses and 8% of GPs do this directly without any assessment. It is relevant therefore that practice nurses understand how to use the auriscope to examine patients and to add quality, effectiveness and safety to ear syringing.

To perform the examination:

- make sure that the batteries are fully charged
- select a large speculum, which will fit comfortably in the ear
- hold the auriscope like a pen in the dominant hand, with the wrist resting against the patient's head. This is particularly relevant for children who may move suddenly and this position will support the ear, and prevent the speculum from digging in
- ask the patient to tilt the head in the opposite direction to the ear being inspected
- for adults gently pull the pina upwards and backwards to straighten the auditory meatus. For children the pina needs to be pulled downwards and out from the body, as the canal is already straight
- insert the speculum slightly down and forward.

Once the speculum is positioned, the ear canal should be inspected for redness, swelling, wax, lesions, scaling, discharge and foreign bodies. Expect to visualise minimal wax, a uniform pink colour and hairs in the outer part of the canal. Inspect the tympanic membrane for its translucent pearly grey colour and any signs of perforation, also for the landmarks of the ossicles, for their contour. Knowing what to look for is essential in assessing the ear and some common findings have been summarised in *Table 4.2*.

Using a vaginal speculum

Women often expect that nurses will have a better appreciation of their feelings and this perception often leads women to seek practice nurses for any form of gynaecological examination or investigation. Most procedures, such as taking a smear or vaginal swab will necessitate practice nurses using a Cusco's speculum, and many women fear this examination believing it to be painful, embarrassing or unpleasant. It is important, therefore, that practice nurses understand how to use the speculum effectively, to obtain the desired results and cause as little discomfort as possible.

Table 4.2: Conditions of the ear

Findings	Causes
Perforated eardrum.	A traumatic blow, loud blast, chronic infection, poking objects into the ear.
Fluid in the middle ear which may also contain bubbles.	Chronic obstruction of the Eustachion tube, due to catarrh. In children this may be adenoid enlargement. Air in the ear which is usually absorbed cannot be replaced.
Red bulging pink eardrums, landmarks impossible to see.	Acute otits media.
Dull, textureless and retracted membrane. Malleus handle is prominent. Fluid level may be visible with bubbles. Colour depends on fluid: yellowish to grey.	Glue ear (secretory otitis media).
Bilateral, non-bulging pink eardrums in children.	Viral infection.
Ear swollen, inflamed, tender to touch with possible crusting and secretions.	Otitis externa.
Bleeding from ear.	Head injury or a ruptured eardrum.

Ideally the patient needs to lie on her back, in an M-shaped position, with her knees bent and feet apart resting on the couch. Performing a speculum examination is an invasion into a person's private territory, which can be threatening, and a powerful, primitive signal of dominance. It is important to cover the patient with a blanket in a way that allows for minimal exposure and maintains dignity. The patient needs to feel involved with what is happening and permission should be sought before starting. Patients also need to be reassured that the procedure will be carried out as gently as possible and encouraged to say if they feel any discomfort.

Select an appropriate sized speculum to suit the patient. It is not always easy to judge this first time, but it is better to choose one that is too long rather than too short as it is better not to insert it all, than change it. The speculum should be warmed to body temperature under the tap. This will also help with insertion, but if necessary a water-based lubricant could be applied. If a smear is to be taken, lubricant should only be applied to the sides and not the tip as this may interfere with cytological readings. The external genitalia should be inspected for sores, genital warts or any unusual characteristics and then the labia should be gently separated with one hand. Insert the closed blades along with the axis of the introitus and, when halfway, rotate them gently through to 90°. Matching the anatomic angle of the vagina press the speculum upward until the cervix is in view and then manipulate the blades a little further into the vagina as far as it will go, which is usually the whole length of the blades. With a deliberate action open the speculum fully tilting it slightly to expose the cervix well between the blades. The cervix may be difficult to locate and some simple tips have been highlighted in *Table 4.3*.

The blades can now be locked into position using the thumb-screw although this is not always necessary depending on the procedure or individual experience. Once the cervix is in full view inspect it for any signs of abnormalities (*Table 4.4*).

The cervix lies in the midline and any deviation from this may indicate a pelvic mass, uterine adhesions or pregnancy. If the cervix protrudes down more than 3cm this may indicate signs of a uterine prolapse.

Inform the patient before removing the speculum, unlocking it and gently rotating it during the withdrawal in order to inspect the vaginal walls for colour, secretions, bleeding, nodules or swelling. Care should be taken to avoid pinching the vaginal mucosa and pubic hair and the cervix needs to be clear before allowing the blade to close automatically. Dispose of the speculum in cold water, which will make it easier to clean in hot soapy water later on. There is evidence to imply that there is a danger of poor hygiene practices in GP surgeries and that some nurses are ignorant of correct sterilising techniques (Cour, 1995). Boiling instruments is not reliable and they should be sterilised in an autoclave for a minimum of 15 minutes at 121°C and after cooling left covered up.

Table 4.3: Common problems in locating the cervix

Problem	Remedy
A very deep cervix (this may sometimes be if patient is very tall, or big built).	Use a Winterton speculum which has extra long blades.
Uterus at an angle.	This may be due to the cervix being retroverted and in the anterior wall, this may be overcome by asking the patient to put her hands under her buttocks or to raise her pelvis. It may also help to ask the patient to half sit-up resting on her elbows. If the cervix points into the posterior wall because the uterus is very antroverted it may be helpful if the patient presses down with her hands over her lower abdomen. Upward and downward searching movements with the speculum may find the cervix or trying the patient in the left lateral position.
Prolapsed vaginal wall falls into the field.	Use a latex finger of a glove, with the closed end cut off as a sheath, over the speculum. The speculum will open stretching the rubber, which will keep the vaginal wall away.
Only tight vaginal wall is seen.	This is usually due to the speculum being incorrectly inserted into the posterior fornix and it may be corrected by easing the speculum forwards and asking the patient to cough.
The speculum causes too much pain to be opened well into the vagina.	This may be due to the fact that the patient has a vaginal infection, if discharge is seen it may be necessary to take a swab and then take the smear after treatment. Peri- and post-menopausal women often suffer with drying and thinning of the vagina and this may cause problems. A smaller speculum could be tried with the use of more lubricant or a short two–six-week course of hormonal vaginal cream or pessaries may be beneficial before a further attempt. Preparations should not be used, however, 24 hours before a smear.

Table 4.4: Characteristics of the cervix

The cervix may:

Appear normal	The cervix should be pink with colour evenly distributed. The os in a nulliparous woman is small, while in a multiparous woman it is usually a horizontal slit.
Appear red	The reasons may be: * Physiological. If the squamocolumnar epithelium is outside the os, this may be visible as a symmetric red circle around the os, know as an ectopy * Pathological. The redness may be due to infection indicating the need for full microbiological investigation.
Have associated appearances	This may be due to: discharge; cysts (nabothian cysts are retention cysts of the endocervical glands and are normal); polyps; vesicles/herpes; ulcers/herpes/syphilis; raised irregular areas/ malignant; white patches/cobblestone appearance/ cervicitis or carcinoma; warts.

Palpation

Palpation follows inspection and involves the use of touch to gather information about the position, shape, size, consistency and mobility of organs or masses. Palpation will also determine the extent of tenderness, site of pain, presence of pulses and temperature of the skin. Different parts of the hands and fingers are better for specific types of palpation (*Table 4.5*).

Table 4.5: Areas of the hand used in palpation

Area	To detect
Back of the hand	Temperature changes.
Surface of the fingers and finger tips	Texture, size, position, consistency, fluid, crepitus, forms such as a mass.
Ulnar surface of the hand and fingers	Vibration, such as the thrill of a heart murmur.

It is helpful to develop a logical sequence to palpation and the point is to acquire an approach that is useful and practical and produces the desired results. The patient should also remain covered except for the area being palpated.

There are specific techniques to palpation which may be either light or deep and this is determined by the amount of pressure applied (*Table 4.6*).
Light palpation should always be performed first as deep pressure can dull the sense of touch. Touch is the first approach to invasion of the patient's body and therefore should be undertaken gently and with respect. Nurses are in an ideal situation to include palpation into their practice, as it is strongly associated with nursing, singling it out from other health care disciplines (Benor, 1996). Touch can be therapeutic and Major (1981) believed that the outcome of the touched can be affected by status of the one touching, eg. the white coat syndrome where authority confers a therapeutic touch. Palpitation offers an opportunity not only to examine the patient, but also in communication as receptivity is enhanced and care may be initiated.

Table 4.6: Types of palpation	
Light palpation	* use the dominant hand parallel to the body's surface * use the palmar surface of the fingertips with fingers together * press downward, moving the hand to depress the area 1cm or less * to distinguish size and shape of masses, push down several times rather than holding the fingers down.
Deep palpation	* instruct patient to breathe deeply * rest the palm of the dominant hand and use fingertips together to palpate * rest hand during inspiration and increase depth of palpation with expiration * depress area to depth of 4cm or more.
Bimanual palpation (this may be used when deep palpation is difficult, eg. due to obesity)	* use one hand on top of the other and undertake the general principles of deep palpation * use one hand to support or elevate an organ, eg. the kidney, while the other hand palpates it.

Issues regarding breast examination and palpation

Walker (1995a) points out that breast examination is one of the most common types of physical examination in which a practice nurse may be involved. A great deal of panic was caused following a joint letter sent by the Chief Medical Officer and the Chief Nursing

Officer, Yvonne Moores, recommending that breast examination should not be promoted as a screening procedure (DoH, 1998a). Calman advised that palpation of the breast by doctors and nurses should not be included as part of routine health screening, as women are more likely to find breast lumps themselves and that the effectiveness of breast self-examination in reducing the mortality from breast cancer has never been consistently demonstrated. While the letter advised that breast examination should not be delegated to nurses in the primary care setting it recognises that nurses, such as those with specialist training in breast care units, should perform this skill. It is arguable that many practice nurses will have specialist training in physical examination and remain as competent as others in this ability, particularly ANPs and nurse practitioners.

Nurses who are unsure of what to do but feel that they are trained sufficiently and are competent and willing to undertake breast examination, need to consider that if a patient comes to them with a breast problem or a suspected lump, they have a duty of care to that patient and should act in the patient's best interests.This is particularly relevant in the circumstances where many nurses are now having their referrals accepted by consultants or breast care units (in some patients can refer themselves). This duty includes both acts and omissions on their part and if they choose not to employ the skill they have this may cause patients delay in care, more worry and even deny them the service they really want.

In order to establish if there has been a breach of duty it is necessary to determine the standard of care expected of the professional in that set of circumstances (Dimond, 1997). Practice nurses need to reflect what standard patients expect from them, particularly as patients are aware that they used this skill before and teach patients how to examine themselves now.

Practitioners are the ones who must ultimately determine their boundaries, and the standard of care provided by health care professionals is judged in the light of current knowledge and advice. The nurse would need to be in a position of explaining and justifying any decision taken as being in the best interests of the patient. In considering the guidelines nurses must consider what Stern (1995) points out: that guidelines can deny the importance of clinical discretion and that until they become rules, it is unlikely that acting upon a guideline *per se* would succeed in court. The NHS Executive (1996) highlights that guidelines can only assist the practitioner and cannot be used to mandate, authorise or outlaw treatment.

Breast examination

Knowing the technique of breast examination is essential for all practice nurses, whether to use it within their role or to obtain appropriate information in order to teach breast awareness. Whatever the scenario, it is important to first obtain a full history from the patient (*Table 4.7*).

Table 4.7: History	
Age — incidence of cancer increases with age.	
Past history — date of last mammogram/ultrasound. Results of previous tests.	
Past history of breast disease — operations, biopsies.	
Family history of breast disease — which relatives and type of disease and outcome.	
Symptom	**Consider**
Tumour	* when first found * changes that were first noticed * location and characteristics * any changes with cycle * nipple changes.
Nipple discharge	* spontaneous or induced * amount and character * when first noted * related to pregnancy or not * taking oral contraceptives or not * breast-feeding.
Pain or tenderness	* in one or both breasts * present all the time or cyclical * type of pain and its character (dull, sharp).

The first part of the breast examination is to inspect the breasts in three positions, observing both breasts before, during and after each manoeuvre.

1. With the patient seated and arms at her sides, look for the size, contour, shape, venous pattern and surface texture of the breasts. Inspect for appearance of the skin whether red, ulcerated or thickened, the skin should be smooth with an uninterrupted contour. A leather puckered appearance like orange skin — peau d'orange — indicates oedema caused by blocked lymph nodes. Note the nipples for any signs of deviation, retraction, inversion (other than longstanding) or discharges, which may present as pus, clear, bloody or milky.

2. With the patient's arms over her head as this elevates the pectoral fascia. If a tumour with fibrosis is present the breast tissue may adhere to it and any overlying skin, causing disruption of the shape or position of the breast or nipple.
3. With the patient's hands pressed against her hips or with palms pressed together across the level of her chin. This contracts the pectoral muscles and elevates the breast. In this position a tumour may cause dimpling.

If the patient has large breasts a fourth position is helpful:

4. Ask the patient to bend forward from the waist with her chin up and arms stretched out in front. If a tumour is present this position can show up any asymmetry or retraction.

Palpation follows inspection and this is best performed with the patient in the supine position and with the arms raised above the head to flatten the breast and expose the axilla. Palpation should be performed slowly using the flat of the fingers to compress the tissue by gently pushing forward towards the chest wall. Use a pattern to examine every inch of the breast and axillary tail. The Tail of Spence is an important area as most malignancies occur in the upper outer quadrant. The pattern could be either spiral, using four quadrants, wheel spoke or clock face. Pressure should be firm enough to obtain a good sense of feel to the tissue beneath. Whatever the method, start with light palpation and then move on to a deeper palpation and finish by examining the tissue below the nipple. If discharge is suspected compress the nipple gently between the finger and thumb, or ask the patient to, and if discharge appears send it for culture and sensitivity or cytopathology if indicated.

It is advisable to develop a personal routine and technique that starts and finishes at a fixed point to make sure that all parts of the breast have been palpated. Palpate each breast in turn, not forgetting to examine the armpits and each clavicle for swollen glands. If the patient has a problem in one breast, examine the other breast first to gain an idea of comparison. If a lump is found note the size, location, shape, consistency, tenderness, deliation of borders and mobility.

Bimanual examination

Tunnadine (1992) points out that the vaginal examination can offer the, 'moment of truth' for women with gynaecological problems. Pelvic examination is very much a part of the practice nurse role, whether to exclude pelvic pathology or simply to locate a difficult cervix prior to a smear. The positioning of the patient is the same as explained previously for taking a smear.

The examination itself begins by inserting the lubricated tip of the gloved index and middle fingers of the dominant hand into the vaginal opening to about 5cm, gently pressing downward, then waiting for the patient to relax her muscles. Gradually insert the length of the fingers into the vagina feeling round the vaginal wall for any cysts, nodules or growths. The vagina should feel smooth, but not tender. Finally, the fingers should rest at the position of the vaginal vault and the cervix should then be felt by running the fingers around its circumference. The cervix normally feels like the tip of the nose, firm and smooth. Move the cervix from side to side 1–2cm in each direction, observing the patient for any signs of discomfort. Painful cervical movement is an indication of acute pelvic inflammatory disease and will need further investigation.

Next feel for the uterus by using the palmar surface of the 'abdominal ' hand midway between the umbilicus and the symphysis pubis, pressing downward. Place the intravaginal fingers deep in the posterior fornix and lift the uterus towards the 'abdominal' fingers using a steady pressure. The idea is to try to bring the two hands together with the uterus in-between. Using a side-to-side motion with the 'vaginal' fingers, the uterus should be assessed for its size, shape, consistency and position (anteverted, anteflexed, mid-position, retroverted or retroflexed).

Follow through to palpate the ovaries and fallopian tubes by moving the 'abdominal' hand to the right side, above the pubic hairline and the intravaginal fingers into the right lateral fornix. Palpate the area by pressing downward with the 'abdominal' hand and upward with the intravaginal fingers. By gently rocking backwards and forwards with the fingers of both hands in opposite directions, the ovaries will be swept over between the fingers. Then move to the left side and repeat the procedure. Normally the ovaries are only palpable at certain times during the menstrual cycle and are therefore often not felt. It is not always normal to feel the ovaries in the postmenopausal woman, but if this is the case this may be an indication of clinical pathology. The ovaries should feel firm, smooth and almond shaped and no other structures except for possibly the round ligaments should be felt.

Percussion

Percussion involves the method of using a finger of one hand as a striking surface and a finger of the other as the hammer to produce vibration and subsequent sound waves. The degree of percussion tones varies according to how the sound waves travel through density of tissue (4–6cm deep) in the body. Normally, the more compact the tissue, the quieter and shorter the tone. There are five sounds: flatness, dullness, resonance, hyper-resonance and tympany (*Figure 4.1*).

Figure 4.1: Percussion notes and sounds

AREA	TISSUE	TONE	INTENSITY	SOUND
	Most dense			
Muscle, full bladder, bone thigh, liver, spleen	▲	Flatness	Soft	Very dull, non-musical
		Dullness	Medium	Thudlike, non-musical
Healthy lung		Resonance	Loud	Hollow, somewhat musical
Emphysematous (lung tissue)		H y p e r - resonance	Very loud between resonance and tympany	Boomlike, musical
Gastric air bubble intestines	▼	Tympanic	Loud	Drumlike, musical, with rich over tones
	Least dense			

Percussion will determine if the tissue is air-filled by being loud, or fluid-filled by being less loud and over solid areas, by being soft. Direct percussion will determine tenderness by tapping the body with one or more finger of one hand over the body. The technique of indirect percussion is performed as follows:

1. Place the non-dominant hand with the fingers slightly spread out on the area to be percussed.
2. Only the middle finger should rest firmly on the body the other fingers should not touch the surface.

3. Use the tip of the middle finger of the other hand to sharply tap the middle finger resting on the body, between the fingernail and distal joint.
4. Use the lightest blow that will produce sound and keep the forearm stationary producing a rapid tap that originates from the wrist.
5. Limit strokes to three or less in each area of equal force.
6. Percuss one place several times to interpret the tone, then move around listening to the sound change.

Learning to distinguish the different sounds requires experience. It can help to practice on a partially full carton of fruit juice, listening for the sound change as the fluid is found.

Auscultation

Auscultation is the process of listening for sounds produced by the body. Direct auscultation involves using the unaided ear, listening for sounds such as wheeze or nasal congestion. With indirect auscultation sounds from the heart, blood vessels, lungs and stomach are heard using a stethoscope and can be described in terms of their timing, intensity (loudness), pitch (high or low), duration (long or short) and quality (rumbling, blowing or musical). The funnel-shaped open bell of the stethoscope has a natural frequency and is used to detect low-pitched sounds such as heart murmurs. This should be applied evenly and lightly to the skin using enough pressure to seal the edges. The rigid diaphragm has a frequency of around 300Hz and will detect high-pitched sounds, such as those found in the lung and faint sounds such as friction rubs, crepitus and heart sounds. To recognise how crepitus in the lung sounds, practitioners should try listening to the sound of their own hair crunched between the finger and thumb of one hand, as this produces a similar sound.

Effective auscultation needs a systematic approach, moving from one area of the body to another, comparing the sound heard on corresponding areas. Closing the eyes may help to focus the sound and prevent distraction from other stimuli. Sounds should be isolated concentrating on one sound at a time in each location, listening specifically to identify its characteristics (*Table 4.9*)

As Walker (1995b) highlights, auscultation is a difficult art and requires practice and experience. It can be useful to practice on willing colleagues, as concentrating on the normal sounds first should make detection of any deviation from this easier.

Table 4.9: Basic identifying sounds

	Finding	Characteristics	Possible cause
The Lungs	Fine crackles	Soft, high in pitch, very brief	Asthma, chronic bronchitis
	Coarse crackles	Louder, lower in pitch and not so brief	
	Wheezes	High in pitch with a hissing quality	
	Rhonchi	Low in pitch with a snoring quality	
	Stridor	Wheeze heard on inspiration only	Obstruction of airway in the neck
	Pleural rub	Creaking, grating sound with respiratory movements	Inflamed pleural surface
The Heart	First and second heart sound	Sounds like 'lub-dub'	Normal
	Third heart sound heard in diastole	Sound like Ken-**tuc**-ky	Early signs of congestive heart failure
	Fourth heart sound before the first heart sound	Sounds like **Ten**-nes-see	Occurs in myocardial infarction
	Prolonged extra sounds heard during systole or diastole (murmurs)	Harsh, blowing	Possibly innocent Caused by diseased valves

Advanced health assessment

To illustrate how the process of examination is incorporated into advanced practice assessment the following case study is presented of an actual case managed by an advanced nurse practitioner in general practice (Prince, 1999). This study highlights how the ANP used the consultation to provide advice, guidance, treatment and health promotion. It reflects the ANP's ability to use the skills presented in *Chapter 3* and is a good example of effective implementation of the hypothetical – deductive model involved in critical thinking discussed in the following chapter.

Case study

The following case focuses on a young nine-year-old child, Wendy, who was brought to the surgery by her mother. She had a rash, which covered her chest, abdomen and legs the day before, but when she came to the surgery it was much paler and not so extensive, covering her upper back, forearms and legs.

History of presenting complaint

Wendy had complained of a sore throat for three to four days and her throat hurt when she swallowed. She had developed a pain in her right ear, which had started that morning which she described as throbbing. The pain was there all the time but it was helped by paracetamol. She did not complain of pain anywhere else.

Background/past history

Wendy is generally a healthy young lady who rarely visits the surgery. She has a history of asthma for which she takes a becotide inhaler 200mg twice daily and salbutamol inhaler when required. Her asthma appears to be well controlled, although her mother was worried that Wendy had not attended the clinic for two years, but after reassurance, she was advised to make an appointment for Wendy in the near future. Wendy had suffered two previous attacks of acute otitis media for which she had been treated with amoxycillin. She had no allergies and was up-to-date with her immunisations, including measles/mumps/rubella.
Hypothesis:
Non-specific viral rash and acute otitis media.
Differential diagnosis:
Meningitis, measles, rubella, mastoiditis, boil in ear canal, inflammation of temporomandibular joint and otitis externa.

Testing of hypothesis by:

Further history
On questioning Wendy it was found that she had no other complaints of pain, for example, a headache. The rash was now not so prominent but it was still a little itchy. Mum said that she had been using calamine lotion to relieve the itchiness, but she was a little worried because she had noticed that it was out of date. Again she was reassured that no harm had been done and that the calamine must have helped even though it was out of date. She said that Wendy had felt 'off colour' for a few days the previous week. She explained Wendy's weepiness as a reaction to the fact that Wendy's older brother had been admitted to hospital for an emergency appendicectomy operation and although he was

all right she was still worried. She had no cough and she was sleeping through the night.

Examination

Wendy walked into the consulting room holding her Mum's hand. She preferred to stand next to her mother rather than sit down and she looked pale with tear-stained eyes, but she responded readily to friendly questioning. She smiled and nodded shyly as attempts were made to put her at her ease. Her neck did not appear swollen and inspection of her mouth with a good light source revealed inflamed mucosa of the nasopharynx, her tonsils were not swollen. Her gums and buccal membrane were pink and healthy and her teeth were clean and intact.

Both ears were examined, the pinna first of all. Both looked healthy with no inflammation. Palpation around both ears, ie. the mastoid bone and the tragus did not produce pain. There was no visible discharge from either ear. Inspection with an auriscope showed the left ear canal to be healthy and the drum shiny, however, the right ear was dry with an inflamed ear canal, and the drum was inflamed but intact.

She had a good range of movement of her neck and was able to attempt to put her chin on her chest quite easily with no neck stiffness. Palpation of her neck did not reveal any swollen glands. The rash blanched readily.

Consideration of differential diagnoses

The signs of meningitis are fever accompanied by headache, neck stiffness and some times a petechial rash (Donaldson and Donaldson, 1983). This condition can therefore be excluded by the fact that Wendy did not have a headache or neck stiffness and her rash blanched easily when pressed.

Measles is sometimes identifiable by the presence of Koplik's (white) spots on the buccal membrane and is usually accompanied by a cough and a maculopapular rash. Rubella is characterised by a fine macular rash and enlargement of the posterior cervical and occipital glands (Donaldson and Donaldson, 1983). The fact that Wendy had been vaccinated against measles, mumps and rubella should not automatically rule out any of these infections from the differential diagnosis because a small percentage of children vaccinated against these diseases do not seroconvert. Vaccination does mean less chance of contracting these infections and the examination revealed none of the signs, which characterise the disease, so they were ruled out from the diagnosis.

Otitis externa and boils of the external auditory canal cause pain due to swelling and narrowing of the canal. Pressing on the tragus anteriorly to the ear causes pain if either of these conditions are present (Browning, 1982). Wendy had no tenderness when this area was gently palpated. Similarly, if mastoiditis has developed there will be pain and tenderness over the mastoid bone (Browning, 1982). Wendy did not demonstrate this symptom on examination so all these conditions can be excluded from the differential diagnosis.

The temporomandibular joint is in such close proximity to the ear that inflammation of this joint presents as otalgia. The commonest cause of temporomandibular joint pain is badly fitting dentures (Browning, 1982). Wendy did not wear dentures!

Confirmed diagnosis

Acute otitis media is a bacterial infection, which causes pain as long as the eardrum stays intact. Pain only subsides with rupture of the tympanic membrane allowing release of pus. Wendy's right drum was intact but inflamed, therefore examination confirmed the original hypothesis of acute otitis media. The rash was fading and did not bear any of the characteristics of specific infections so the diagnosis of non-specific was was maintained.

Management

Wendy was treated with Amoxil syrup125ml three times a day for the acute otitis media and advised to continue with the paracetamol for relief of the pain. She was encouraged to drink plenty of clear fluids and she was advised to contact the surgery or come back if the symptoms did not improve. Both were asked if they had any worries and if they were happy with the management suggested. Wendy's mum mentioned the fact that she was worried about a recent outbreak of meningitis in the area. She was reassured concerning the absence of signs and symptoms of meningitis and the opportunity was taken to offer advice on the signs and symptoms such as neck stiffness, headache and petechial rash and what to do if she suspected this condition in any of her family.

This consultation was not clear-cut, as is usually the case in general practice. While Wendy presented with a rash, by using examination skills it was possible to determine that she also had an ear infection. Her background history of asthma needed further follow up and Wendy's mother's true anxiety seemed to stem around fears of meningitis for which she needed information, reassurance and guidance. Management of patient problems are manifold and not based solely on medical treatment. Through effective interviewing skills and physical examination the ANP was able to offer a comprehensive, holistic consultation and provide the kind of care practice nursing is all about.

5

Critical thinking in general practice

*'Would you tell me, please, which way I ought to
go from here?' 'That depends a good deal on
where you want to get to', said the Cat.*
Alice in Wonderland, Lewis Carroll

The ability to think critically is an important aspect of the practice
nurse role and its capacity to function successfully within the climate
of general practice. Practice nurses need to be competent in their
thinking processes in order to evaluate client problems, recognise
health problems and provide accurate solutions. Decision-making is
complex and practice nurses have to be equipped with the
intellectual skills to gather and analyse complex amounts of data and
later process it into alternatives made from precise deliberation and
judgement. Discriminative thinking will also depend on the
professional artistry of individuals and the way it is processed and
interpreted will be different among practitioners because of their
contrasting levels of skills, knowledge and experience. Within
advanced practice, the advanced nurse practitioner (ANP) works
with tremendous amounts of information, using high levels of
critical thought to analyse problems from diverse perspectives to
reach a high order of synthesis, understanding and choice. This
characteristic way of thinking by ANPs has forms and patterns to it,
which are useful to explore in order to highlight and clarify the range
of knowledge held by ANPs. This, in turn, should also help those
wishing to develop their abilities or provide *raison d'être* behind the
care necessary for effective practice.

What is meant by the term critical thinking?

Although there has been many definitions of critical thinking within
the literature (*Table 5.1*), it has only recently been addressed to
nursing.
   There is widespread acknowledgement that nurses should use
some form of structured thinking to direct their actions. Schaefer

(1974) identified three phrases to the process; deliberation, judgement and choice. There is a high degree of subjectivity to judgement in practice and how it is made will be dependent upon the type, level and breadth of theoretical knowledge and practice that influences it. For Schaefer the greater the deliberation and judgement the greater the decision will be. This emphasises the importance of comprehensive rationalising, analysing and thinking abilities. Implicit within this thinking is the notion of weighing up ideas and assumptions in the form of logical arguments, and there is a clear relationship between thoughts and the intellect. Critical thinking itself is distinct from any other forms of thinking, such as daydreaming, because it requires a form of purposeful action and evaluation, it is also retrospective because information is needed prior to its inception. The overall outcome of critical thinking is to reach a solution to a problem or, if not, to have a greater understanding of it.

Table 5.1: Definitions of critical thinking

Source	Definition
Beyer (1984)	A combination of problem-solving and basic thoughts.
Burnard (1990)	The ability to generate options and possibilities and to discriminate intellectually, to be creative and to identify new ideas.
Ennis (1985)	Reflective and reasonable thinking that is focused on what to believe and do.
Facione and Facione (1994)	The cognitive engine driving the processes of knowledge, development and clinical judgement in nursing.
Garver (1986)	A developmental progression from concrete to formal thought.
Halpern (1989)	Purposeful, reasoned and goal-directed thinking.
Jones and Brown (1991)	A complex cognitive process, requiring application of higher order thinking to decision-making in practice.
Landis and Michael (1981)	Awareness of a problem situation and the evaluation of numerous decisions prior to action that may not always solve the problem.
McPeck (1981)	An involvement of scepticism which may give way to acceptance, but considers alternative hypotheses and possibilities before taking truth for granted.
Watson and Glaser (1991)	A composite of attitudes, knowledge and skills.

Within nursing, Bandman and Bandman (1995) suggested that there are several critical thinking functions, including:

- examination of nursing assumptions
- ensuring that inferences are plausible
- corroborations and justification of claims, beliefs, conclusions, decisions and actions
- seeking reasons, criteria and principals to justify judgements
- ability to analyse arguments into premises and conclusions
- making and checking inferences based on data
- evaluating the soundness of conclusions.

Thus, critical thinking involves many intellectual skills within nursing in order to produce and evaluate judgements that relate to quality care. Critical thinking is not something that everyone does, nor is it undertaken in the car on the way home from work. It is a purposeful activity, which needs to be practised. Some people are more adapt at thinking than others and the American Philosophical Association (APA, 1990) provide a list of common attributes they believe to be characteristic of a critical thinker. These are:

- flexible
- open-minded
- customary inquisitive
- confident of reason
- content to reconsider
- well-informed
- fair in evaluation
- clear about matters
- diligent in searching for significant information
- honest in confronting personal prejudices
- disciplined in complexity
- shrewd in making decisions
- sensible in selecting patterns of enquiry
- persistent in obtaining precise results.

Critical thinking can therefore be regarded as a reasoning process, that involves intellectual skills, personal attributes and deliberate activity in order to produce views that can be evaluated into accurate judgements and solutions.

Why do practice nurses need to be critical thinkers?

There seems to be a view that all nurses in general need to be critical thinkers on the grounds that it is of benefit to practice and that this can be liberating (Bandman and Bandman, 1995). Similarly Alfaro-Lefevre (1995) claim that all nurses need critical thinking to produce sound clinical judgements.

For practice nurses critical thinking is the hallmark of effective practice and the requirement for being competent and skilful. Jones and Brown (1991) see it as being essential to true autonomy — as many practice nurses work with professional freedom, it is integral to being able to practice soundly and safely. Practice nurses need to use critical thinking effectively to provide diagnosis for patient complaints. They are often the first line contact for patients presenting with, and needing identification of rashes, infections, lumps, discharges, coughs and colds. Diagnosis was previously the sole remit of medicine and its inheritance has left many nurses in doubt as to having authority to acquire it. This is attributable no doubt to lingering influences of past subservience to medicine. However, few would question, the mechanic who specifies a problem with a car, or a teacher who identifies a child with dyslexia. Today, diagnosis is part of the modern practice nurse role and by implementing high levels of critical thinking and professional judgement, practice nursing will come further into its own as a distinct discipline and take on more of an independent place alongside the activities of GPs.

The role of practice nurses has expanded into the realms of physical health assessment. This role, which has been specifically looked at in *Chapter 4*, requires an analytical ability and skill that depends upon accurate critical thinking and reasoning to be successful. Within the current general practice climate of cost implication and justification, professional and clinical judgements will have to be made in a rational, logical and coherent way if they are to be both credible and accepted. Critical thinking will also be important to develop and articulate strategies relevant to Government policy and provide answers to today's increasingly complex health care environment.

People generally understand what it means to think but few can describe how thinking occurs, particularly in nursing. Through understanding the mental processes and strategies that solve problems it is possible for practice nurses to improve clinical reasoning skills and develop self-awareness related to individual thinking. According to Arons (1985), critical thinking can be cultivated by practitioners raising questions; probing assumptions; being aware of gaps in information; as well as discriminating between observation and evidence. These techniques are relevant for academic writing and for nurses who wish to obtain postgraduate qualifications, as critical thinking and analysis is central to course work, discussions and debates. In turn, the knowledge gained from studying with an inquiring, open mind, sensitive to multiple perspectives, will help to integrate a theory-based practice which reflects nursing at its best (Edwards, 1998). Embodying the art of critical thinking through expert practice will also be a step forward for practice nurses who wish to become ANPs.

Models of thinking and reasoning

Critical thinking is a method of problem-solving for which the process of making decisions is integral. The skills involved in good decision-making are central to the overall competencies of nurses, particularly practice nurses, as they underpin most of their work through consultations with patients which involves giving correct diagnosis, treatment or advice. Practice nurses, unwittingly, use a variety of models to ask patients questions and reach conclusions (Paniagua, 1997). The most frequent method used is probably that of decision analysis, which involves accumulating segments of information, making choices from a number of alternatives and recombining them into a logical chain. The passage from the first question, to the final firm conclusion, is comprised of a sequence of decision events. The outcomes of these events have a significant effect on the actual course future thoughts will take. The resulting model can be illustrated in the form of a decision tree. *Figure 5.1* shows a decision tree for the diagnosis of vaginal bleeding.

Within the tree each branching point represents a location where another competing decision has to be made depending upon the outcome.

This model is useful in critical thinking as it forces the decisions that need to be made, while simultaneously answering the possible consequences and uncertainty for each decision. This method of thinking is effective in helping nurses to synthesise all the possible information and to decide upon the best estimate diagnosis or answer from all the factors involved.

Figure 5.1: An example of a decision tree

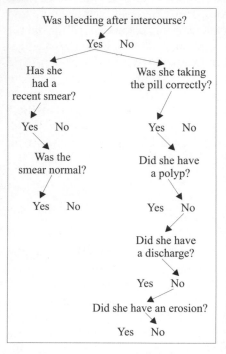

A further model used by practice nurses is that of the hypothetical-deductive model, which involves the forming of a hunch or tentative hypothesis, and then searching for further information or cues presented by the patient to confirm or disprove it (*Figure 5.2*).

This really is a process that works backwards and involves forming clusters of cues that match patterns, and gradually the search becomes more focused into fewer probable diagnoses.

Within this model the nurse will be making and matching patterns from uncertainty, gathering information, making sense of it and giving it various weighting to match it with already gained knowledge based on previous experience. This method can lead nurses into problems, as it is very dependent on the practitioner's perception and understanding. If perception is guided by stereotyping a prejudiced mind can block further communication and thought processes needing open judgement.

The information processing model is an alternative model implemented by practice nurses, which consists of a sequence of questions to the patient through IF-THEN paired inferential statements or rules. One example of a rule might be IF the patient is excessively thirsty THEN this might be a sign of diabetes. The knowledge gained triggers off further rules held within the individual store of knowledge, eg. IF the patient is a diabetic THEN this will show in the blood sugar level. The nurse can operate using a large number of rules obtained from past experiences and learning stored with the memory.

There are no rules in deciding which model to use, and often practice nurses use several models together or interchangeably. The frequency and pattern of using models seems to vary, as does the individual whim. Models, however, need to be used constructively and purposefully, and this can only be achieved by understanding the processes behind clinical thinking and being aware of one's own store of information and individual skill in reasoning.

Figure 5.2: Presenting problem — an eight-year-old child appears to have red spots on her chest

Tentative hypothesis?	Confirmed?	Disproved?
Chickenpox	Spots itchy, do not disappear when pressed	No history of being in contact with infection. No characteristic blisters
	Need to define further hypothesis	
If no blisters but itchy? Scabies	Child appears well, spots itchy, do not disappear when touched	No revealing blue tracks, no rash on back of hands, rash not symmetrical
	Need to define further hypothesis	
If no characteristics of childhood illness? Allergic reaction	Itchy rash, child well, no signs or symptoms of childhood infection. Mother says child ate pineapple for the first time two days ago, the rash appeared that same night.	Hypothesis confirmed

How experts think in action

For experts, knowledge accrues over time and this specialised knowledge and accumulated experience lay the foundations for expert thinking. As clinical knowledge accumulates, many patient's problems are noted and imprinted within the memory. Impressions are gradually made about what patients say, patterns of illness, distinguishing and common features of conditions and interesting or different presentation of problems which come to mind as patients are seen with similar concerns. Eventually, experts store vast information based on memorable cases which can be quickly accessed or activated from a cue or signal picked up from a patient. Experts will also use and cross-link multiple cues as opposed to the less experienced, who would be more likely to use single cues to trigger thoughts or even ignore cues which they do not recognise.

Expert nurses, such as ANPs, often have immense, diverse and intricately connected knowledge bases about patients they have seen and the problems that they have presented with.

However, expert thinking involves more than accumulating stores of knowledge, it also includes processing information into meaningful interpretations and decisions. For ANPs, decision- making models will be used more quickly as experts are able to extend their search for cues quickly from a vast range of possibilities, accepting or rejecting cues from complex systems of pattern relationships held within their experience and knowledge store. The more novice nurse will rely on frameworks of rules, guidelines and possibly written templates to understand a situation and make a judgement. The more enriched and accurate the thinking basis, the more likelihood of achieving the dual objective of understanding patients and diagnosing the underlying problems.

When experts are asked how they approach decision-making they often refer to using intuition, and many, such as Benner (1984) draw heavily on the concept as the root of expert decision-making. The experience of making intuitive judgements is disconcerting for those who believe it to be unprofessional or irrational. There seems to be two schools of thought regarding professional decision making: those who believe in a technical and rational approach, and those who believe in artistry and striving for recognition of forms of knowledge outside the realms of empirical science. Views exist that there is a rational basis behind intuition as it could be triggered by some specific — if unconscious — thought rooted in past learning or experience. Intuitive knowing is individual and while it cannot be explained in a tangible manner it is endorsed by many as having a fundamental part to play in skilled decision-making. Benner *et al* (1996) claim that, 'expert practice is characterised by increased intuitive links between seeing the salient issues in the situation and ways of responding to them'. They conclude that expert practice is recognised by mature and practical reasoning, which is accompanied by an intuitive grasp of patient situations. According to Benner, expertise, together with its relevant analytical process, is impossible to define or express in words, as it is dependent upon unconscious intuitive processes embedded in tactic knowledge and know-how.

Rolf (1998) believes that while expert knowledge might be unconscious it does not mean that it is unknowable or an irrational process. He sees it more as a form of testing out hypothesis construction unconsciously and that it therefore has a logical, understandable process, which can ultimately become elevated into consciousness. For Benner, expert practice incorporates intuition that is a form of understanding without a rationale, but for Rolf intuition exists, but has a possible rationale that is not always recognised. It is the contention here that it is possibly a mixture of both depending upon the particular occasion or experience, which comes into play at the time. To put one belief above the other is to deny the cognitive abilities or intuitive nature behind advanced practice, which although not mystical, is certainly a phenomenon that has yet to be explained in terms of western empirical science or knowledge.

Intuition is often difficult to explain, Rolf (1997) believes it is possible to understand it in terms of fuzzy logic and abductivism, this in itself adds an interesting perspective to expert thinking. The concept of abductivism turns logic upside down by beginning with the conclusion and then arguing backwards by using understood principals. Rolf uses the example of the general rule that cars need petrol to go and states that if a car does not go the thinking and conclusion is that it has no petrol. While there are other possibilities that could explain the problem, there is a need to apply personal and general knowledge in order to select the most likely supposition, eg. the car has a new battery and starter motor so these are not the causes of the problem. By combining the logic of these fuzzy rules it is possible to make an estimate on the weighted average and come up with the most likely explanation.

Fuzzy logic has been used in programming computers, using vague and imprecise instructions, such as 'a bit to the right'. The result is that computers can now fly helicopters better than experts by using only one hundred fuzzy rules and weighing them up logically. For Rolfe, generating fuzzy rules into computers is the conceptualisation and verbalisation of expert thinking that cannot be rationally shown. While the knowledge base of ANPs is largely tacit and therefore not easy to put into words, it is often felt that if the expert is mindful of what they are doing, performance will suffer. Dreyfus and Dreyfus (1986) see this in performances such as driving a car which, for experts, is automatic and effortless. Once actions are thought about and done deliberately, such as changing gear, then performance becomes less smooth.

It would appear that expert thinking is a complex process, difficult to pinpoint yet rich in consequences; the deeper, more varied and broader the thinking the greater the possibilities and potentialities.

The knowledge behind critical thinking

In order for nurses to make sense of their practice worlds and to understand the thinking used within them, it is relevant to make sense of knowledge and understand where it comes from. Knowledge is intrinsically interwoven within thinking — without it thinking cannot take place, and if not the end result, then thinking becomes a mere reverie. Carper (1978) identified knowing in relation to nursing within four patterns: empirical, ethical, aesthetic and personal. It is useful to look further into each of these in the attempt to explore individual feelings and perception.

Empirical knowledge – this refers to scientific, technical or factual knowledge, which is gained fundamentally through education, reading and research. It forms the science of nursing which involves using learnt theories and organised facts to describe, explain or predict nursing phenomena. This knowledge is particularly relevant for health assessment, physical examination and making a medical diagnosis.

Ethical knowledge – this applies to knowing right from wrong, from the moral experience acquired during life. For nurses, ethical values may come into conflict with legal or professional demands.

Aesthetic knowledge – this is used here as synonymous with the art of nursing which sits uncomfortably with scientific knowledge. It incorporates the intuitive nature of individual judgement and experience.

Personal knowledge – this is the knowing of oneself and the perception of individual feelings and prejudices. It is also thought of as the knowledge acquired through life experiences, which might be more general than scientifically-based. This type of knowledge is significant in understanding the difference between a novice and an expert, whose personal knowledge will be extensive.

In her work, Benner (1984) identified practical knowledge as an important aspect of knowledge for nurses, particularly for the discretionary judgement behind expert knowledge. This included graded qualitative distinctions, common meanings, assumptions, expectations and sets, paradigm cases and personal knowledge, maxims and unplanned practice. For Benner, nurses will acquire this knowledge as they move through a five-stage sequence of proficiency:

1. Novice
2. Advanced beginner
3. Competent
4. Proficient
5. Expert.

A further pattern of knowing has been identified by Munhall (1993) which, paradoxically, is unknowing. This is based on the premise that nurses can never understand patients on first encounter and by recognising this unknowing, the nurse will remain open and focused on the client's perceptions. For Munhall this is an art that promotes alertness to continual learning and to deny unknowing because of personal satisfaction of performance, is considered to be the most prevailing obstacle to developing expert practice.

There are other suggestions to categorising knowledge such as that of Heath (1998), who included socio-political knowledge which refers to knowing based on social policy, economic and political considerations. While other patterns address the 'how, who and what', this aspect incorporates the element of 'where'.

Framing knowledge can make sense of the reality and foundational principals of professional life, and to understand application to practice, nurses can utilise different questions to identify types of knowledge used (*Table 5.3*).

To understand types of knowledge is to realise the trends, arguments and inner disharmonies within nursing. The current fashion in Britain is to encourage evidence-based practice, utilised from research-based empirical knowledge. Nursing is also concerned with developing its own professional knowledge base, which relies heavily on technical rationality and scientific values. Feminist theorists claim that scientific knowledge is given the highest status and considered as the only legitimate knowledge because it is created by and for male interests, and they have the power to label it as such (Hagell, 1988).

Scientific dependence is in danger of destroying the holistic nature of practice and has little to do with advanced practice, which relates to personal and experiential knowledge gained from unique situations, personality and know-how. Hagell (1988) also believes that science and technology undermine the feminist knowledge within nursing, which involves women's life instinct and the humanness of a relationship. This nursing knowledge incorporates knowledge of people and their health-illness experiences, which has affinity with the skill and acuity of advanced practice in elucidating the world of human activity and the knowledge of human-to-human caring.

Table 5.3: Identification of types of knowledge

Type of knowledge	Explanation of knowledge	Where knowledge is discovered from	Questions acquiring knowledge
Empirical (Carper, 1978)	This is synonymous with using scientific information for the purpose of understanding. Facts do not change and can be easily explained. Relies on theory or abstract principles.	Books, journals, research, audit the media or lectures.	What information did or should inform me?
Ethical (Carper, 1978)	This is knowing what is right from wrong and taking action on it.	Consequences of problems or dilemmas that occur in personal or professional life.	How are my actions influenced by my beliefs?
Personal (Carper, 1978)	This is knowing the self, including feelings and prejudices, in order to respond appropriately.	Confusion worked out from experiences, which relate to specific situations, people and events.	How did I feel at the time?
Aesthetic (Carper, 1978)	This is knowledge that has no rational explanation. It often involves the artistry of nursing. Often worked out unaided and is difficult to understand.	Experiences of using empathy and applying intuition.	How do I know things? What are the consequences of my actions on others and myself?
Nursing/Women's (Hagell, 1988)	This is knowing from life instinct.	The social world and daily construct lived.	What is it that I know and experience?
Socio-political (Heath, 1998)	This is the use of knowledge based on factors influenced by the structure of society.	The effects of social, economic and political policy on identity, situations, culture, people and practices.	Where is my voice heard?

Ethical thinking

Moral reasoning is also fundamental to knowledge and critical thinking, its complexity being tied up within ideas of morality and ethics. The skills of managing ethical and moral dilemmas are reliant upon being able to think critically and to make a choice. Nursing is inherently tied up with the need to arrive at conclusions on which actions are morally preferable, and this places utmost emphasis on being able to interpret issues that are not easily understood or dealt with. For ANPs the ability to think ethically is crucial to their role because of the complexity of their relationships, which will often intensify perspectives and responsibilities. Ethical thinking is facilitated from intellect and objectivity and is more than just following rules or intuition; it concerns deciding what is the correct thing to do. Decision therefore depends on knowing what is meant by correct.

Knowledge of moral philosophies and theories can help to promote an ethical way of thinking and the possible answers from different points of views. As explained by Tschudin (1992):

> *A decision is only ethical if it is based on something firm.*
> *Theories supply that firm ground.*

p. 48

The main approaches to this theory follow the thinking of **deontology** and **consequentialism**. Deontology rests on the premise of a morality that depends upon an individual acting upon certain principles, which are duties, and sees right within the features of an action which is independent of consequences; it has doubts in the ability to predict the future to make decisions. Consequentialism sees right within the good produced as a consequence of an action, and this rests upon weighing up the benefits and disadvantages of these consequences.

Deontology stems from the idea that in order to be moral an individual must always do their duty, and this is without exception and regardless of the consequences. This school of thought can be broken down into whether it is based on rules or not. **Act-deontology** is centred on the belief that each situation is unique and therefore rules cannot be applied and situations and judgements only require that a person is true to themselves in moral situations. **Rule-deontology**, on the other hand, is based on the premise that moral choosing can rest on rules, and these should be followed without exception, regardless of consequences.

The best known advocate of this thinking was Immanuel Kant (1724–1804), and his theory was known as the 'categorical imperative'. Kant claimed that if someone wishes to act morally they need to act as if each circumstance will be the law of the future, and that everyone must be seen as an end in themselves, not as the means, and finally always act as an equal member of a community and legislate for all.

Consequentialism is viewed in terms of good as a result of consequences, a brand of this being **utilitarianism**. Utilitarianism views morality on the goal of happiness and within this there is no inherent right thing to do, and motives are not important, it is the result that counts. The measure is not in duty but cost and benefit. The best known exponents of this were Jeremy Bentham (1748–1832) and John Stuart Mill (1806–1873). Both were exponents of the 'greatest happiness principle' where a person should try to achieve, 'the greatest good, or greatest happiness, of the greatest number.' Mill (1910) also insisted that:

> *Utilitarian standard of what is right in conduct is not the agent's own happiness but that of all considered. As between his own happiness and that of others, utilitarianism requires him to be as strictly impartial as a disinterested and benevolent spectator.*

p. 18

Again, this philosophy is broken down into types of rule acceptance or not. **Act-utilitarianism** does not accept rules, only the balance of action of doing more good over evil. **Rule-utilitarianism** is based not only on personal judgement, but on the obedience to certain rules in order to produce the greatest good.

It is not proposed here that in order to think or behave ethically practitioners need to act precisely in accordance with or subscribe to a particular moral theory. In reality, most actions embrace a mixture of principles, for example, within general practice, the giving of immunisation, which has a potential risk, is based upon the balance of greatest good, through herd immunity. The amount of information given about the actual pain of the injection may also depend upon how far the practitioner feels it is their duty to tell the truth.

Ethical thinking is not based entirely on theoretical knowledge; reasoning must be modified within clinical reality. This knowledge is useful however, in trying to understand different standpoints or in trying to make sense of situations. To make ethical theories more applicable, they also have to be viewed within certain principles, which Tschudin (1992) suggest act like a compass, providing direction rather than an actual road map. The most widely accepted principles are those of:

1. **Autonomy**: This is the ability to make choices and is concerned with control and self-government.
2. **Beneficence:** This is doing good through positive acts. It is strongly connected to the caring perspective within nursing.
3. **Non-maleficience**: This implies to do no harm and as Gillion (1986) points out, encompasses all people, whereas the scope of beneficience is more specific, referring only to a few people. This is a principle implicit to informed consent.
4. **Justice**: This is a notion on being fair, the three types include:
   - to each according to his/her rights
   - to each according to what he/she deserves
   - to each according to his/her needs.

These principles are intrinsically linked to issues of screening and health promotion, which form a major component of the role of practice nursing. The way screening is implemented will influence how much harm and good is applied to individuals. The high levels of anxiety experienced by people participating in many screening programs such as cervical cancer or breast cancer screening may have a harmful knock-on effect on physical health. This outcome is directly opposed to the caring ideology of nursing and above all to do no harm. It is also in conflict with one of the criteria laid down for the viability of screening by Wilson and Jungner (1968), namely that the chance of physical or psychological harm should be less than the chance of benefit.

There are no answers to these dilemmas and nursing actions and interventions will inevitably depend upon each practitioner's individual way of thinking and value systems. Often individuals are unaware of their own mental processes when making ethical decisions (Grundstein-Amado, 1992). There are models to assist in guiding ethical thinking and these can be found in *Table 5.4.*

Table 5.4: Models of ethical decision-making

Grundstein-Amado (1992)	Jameton (1984)	Crisham in Scott (1985)
a) problem perception b) information processing c) identification of the patient's preferences d) identification of the ethical issues	Identify the problem	Massage the dilemma
e) listing of possible alternatives	Gather data	
f) their consequences	Identify options Think the problem through Make a decision	Outline options Review criteria resolution
g) the selection of a chosen course of action.	Act	Act
h) finding its justification	Assess	Look back and evaluate

The ability to utilise effective ethical decision-making skills is fundamental to advanced practice. Reigle (1996) believes it incorporates skills that:

> *Move the resolution or moral dilemmas beyond individual cases towards the cultivation of an environment in which the moral integrity of individuals is respected.*

p. 277

This also requires a high level of thinking in order to facilitate dialogue based on options and optimal solutions, anticipate situations and recognise the subtleties of moral issues.

Self-reflection

It can be seen that in order to create any thought, thinking itself stems from many influences and backgrounds. Descartes (1984) perpetuated the power of thought in his adage, 'I am thinking, therefore I exist', and in thinking what nurses do and how they do it, is the basis for the truth of nursing, advanced practice and the recognition of general practice nursing as a distinct discipline within its own right. Self-reflection is the means of empowering nurses to become fully mindful of their own knowledge, and a way of listening to individual thinking processes before, after and in practice.

Critical reflection upon practice is also a way of developing knowledge further. It can also clarify and enhance the art and value of expert nursing. Emden (1991) claims that it should be the aspiration of all mature nurses to become reflective practitioners by thinking and questioning practice and not taking it for granted.

Thinking about individual practice involves reflection which is deliberate and structured. There have been many models offered for this, such as those by Gibbs (1988), Atkins and Murphy (1994) and Johns (1994). It is not within the remit of this chapter to explain individual models but, in mentioning them, to emphasise the fact that in order to gain knowledge from reflection it has to be a structured process, not just a passive contemplation. The aim of reflection is to learn future actions by acting as a mirror to analyse past and present experiences. Reflection requires thinking about situations in new ways and from different perspectives, assessing problems and recognising options. Reflection also necessitates a willingness to learn about self, individual knowledge and practice. As Fernandez (1997) points out, 'We can only notice something if we pay particular attention to it and we only pay attention if we have some idea where to look' (p. 939).

The capacity to reflect mindfully has been described by Schön (1983) within two practices, 'reflection-in-action', which is the ability to think about the situation as it unfolds, and 'reflection-on-action' which is the retrospective thinking about positive and negative experiences, encounters and situations. It seems inevitable that knowledge will come from many experiences, particularly the understanding of events and perceptions. Van Manen (1990, 1991) suggested further forms of reflection related to nursing, including:

- anticipatory reflection — where different approaches to patient care are considered during first assessment
- active reflection, which is literally thinking continuously
- mindfulness or intentional involvement in immediate clinical situations
- recollective reflection, which is a past event reflection.

Reflective practice is considered essential to the professional artistry of nursing practice as it, 'can engender a flexible approach that moves away from rigid behaviour, and avoids the inherent dangers of an increasingly scientific approach within a caring profession' (Turnbull, 1999). This notion can also be extended to incorporating the art of nursing within medical approaches. Conway (1998) identifies the benefits of using reflection as a means to integrate medical tasks within a nursing framework (*Figure 5.3*). This is particularly pertinent to ANPs where physical examination is an essential component and needs to be used within a holistic nursing focus. Conway goes further to underpin the need for reflection for practice nurses in particular in this aspect for without it:

> *It would be easy, given the nature of the contractual relationships between many practice nurses and GPs, for the nurse's role development to be seen only in terms of acquisition of more and more medical tasks.*

p. 15

Reflection also provides experts with the ability to justify clinical decisions and provide reasoned arguments for action (Rolf, 1998). For Rolf, the reflective practitioner is able to generate knowledge as well as acquire it, which is particularly relevant for nursing, where there is a need to move forward as a profession and actually describe what and how it practices.

In order to accommodate personal reflection, illuminate thinking and understand how thinking can change values, practice and attitudes, many advocate the use of diaries or journals. To be effective, writing needs to be accurate and sufficiently detailed to provide a thorough account of feelings, players, events and circumstances. There is also a need to be honest and self-aware about what is written and to re-examine entries asking questions and making comparisons with clinical situations and practice. The keeping of a journal is also beneficial for political and professional purposes where critical reflection is also a pre-requisite. Writing can become a symbolic expression of thought and a critical thinking tool that can generate knowledge unique to the individual. A further vehicle for acquiring and humanising knowledge is that of story telling. Bowles (1995) argues that today's:

> *Environment alienates nurses from each other and their patients, leaving them emotionally impoverished and distanced from the basic humanity of their craft.*

p. 365

Figure 5.3: The integration of practice nursing within a reflective framework, reproduced by kind permission from Jane Glaze (Conway, 1988)

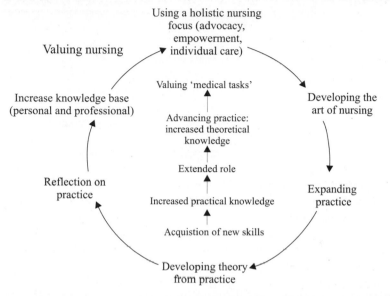

Bowles believes that to be able to listen and utilise stories can be a powerful professional tool to contextualise knowledge and to acquire a deeper understanding of self and others. The process also serves to illustrate lived experience, identify cultural identity, evoke kinship and promote a better understanding of the world of others. The process of narrating often uncovers personal truths, behaviours, and first hand experiences not facilitated by pure thinking or questioning.

Stories or personal accounts of experience can be utilised to educate and investigate practice within formal teaching, writing, clinical supervision, reflection or actual research purposes.

If practice nurses are to value their work and recognise and justify what they have to offer, they need to be able to think critically and utilise the skills that help them to do so. For ANPs the ability to articulate, synthesise and apply rich sources of thinking and knowledge will demonstrate how advanced practice is distinguished. Expert thinking, together with personal and professional knowledge, forms the underpinning of advanced practice, its generation of potential and effectiveness of spontaneous performance. Thinking successfully holds the key to the future of nursing.

6

Embarking on a future role in advanced practice

Change comes from small initiatives which work,
initiatives which initiated become the fashion.
We cannot wait for great visions from great
people, for they are in short supply at the end of
history. It is up to us to light our own small fires
in the darkness.

The Empty Raincoat, Charles Handy

The present is a momentous time for the advanced nurse practitioner (ANP), best epitomised by someone who is ambitious, highly motivated and entrepreneurial. The nursing world and policy makers of today are more in tune with the spirit of pioneers and expert roles. There is a strategic fit with the notion of the ANP and the political ideology of the present government, which promotes nursing leadership, innovation and change. The role, by its very distinction of being non-traditional and thriving on practising autonomously, has the potential towards a career with future, reward and profitable reality. The road to eminence however, is not preordained and will not be easy; success will depend solely on the visions, desires, determination and tenacity of each individual. In order to survive in the community the ANP will also need to understand the many issues and challenges ahead, particularly those that lie embedded within core occupational beliefs and values, power relationships and predominantly the driving forces behind political change.

The years ahead in general practice seem of great promise, as well as great risk, for the ANP.

Changes within primary care

There are going to be fundamental policy changes in the organisation of primary care over the next decade, which will offer many opportunities for practice nurses, particularly those wishing to play a lead role such as ANPs or consultant nurses. Yet change of this magnitude will need a significant shift in the occupational culture, values and beliefs of community nurses in order to realign with the thinking behind this new agenda. The ethos of general practice is now one of change and reorganisation. The White Paper, *The new NHS — modern, dependable* (DoH, 1997), together with the *NHS Plan* (DoH, 2000) seek to modernise the NHS, heavily emphasising inclusion of everyone with a legitimate interest. Opportunities now exist for nurses to become key drivers for change, and for their voices to be heard.

Previously practice nurses had no formal involvement in fund holding, but now this has ended together with the internal market, paving the way for a new ideology that depends on decisions by wider groups of stakeholders. This marks the end of an era and the beginning of change that has already been heralded as the biggest reform of the health service since it was created (Health Service Journal, 1997). The major strategy is for incremental and gradual change, the speed of which is to 'be locally driven' (House of Commons, 1998) and the ANP needs to be there every step of the way.

Planning and commission now lies in the hands of primary care groups (PCGs) expected to cover an area population of around 100,000 people, and nurses have been allocated places on the PCG boards. These PCGs have the opportunity to become future primary care trusts (PCTs), with potentially more power and control over management , provision of services and care. It seems natural that ANPs with their recognition of having enhanced management, leadership and political skills, would fit in well within the fora of PCG boards. The inevitability of ANPs being appointed, however, is not so certain, and as Parkin (1999a) suggests while PCGs may be seen as high performance work teams, there needs to be a major shift in professional perspectives and approaches for future outcomes to be achieved. Success will depend on nurses being able to rethink their roles, work together in partnership breaking down hierarchical structures and developing active involvement rather than passive following.

Marginalisation within PCGs

The Government's intentions for PCGs is to improve the quality of health care by empowering frontline professionals to work together in partnership and co-operation to develop local health care. While it was commendable for the Government to recognise the importance of local-based decisions-making, it is easy to be cynical about its level of conviction in the feasibility of such partnerships. McClure (1995) defined partnership as a, 'particular relationship, encompassing mutual recognition, respect and a degree of equality in status.' In terms of nurse/doctor joint working, to expect this partnership to be assured in many instances is unrealistic.

Partnership on PCG boards will be a challenge for many nurses, both in terms of gaining it and sustaining it. Against this background, nurses who aspire to such places will need to create a new leadership voice for nurses. As highlighted by Antrobus and Kitson (1999), previous nursing leadership has focused on orientating the profession to influence nursing, now they will have to become a vehicle where health and social policy as well as nursing practice can be moulded.

Potential and actual board nurses will also have to challenge the power bases, monopoly and relationships held by GPs under present board design. Despite earlier Government recommendations that boards should not be dominated by individuals or professional groups, GPs have a protected majority of up to seven out of thirteen board places as well as the chair, nurses having only two. GPs were extremely vocal in influencing the configuration of PCGs while nurses remained silent. As remarked by Smith *et al* (1999) perhaps because nurses did not expect much, then they did not get much. The concessions went to GPs who retained their absolute confidence in their 'right' to be at the forefront. As a result, nurses can become marginalised and GPs, if they wish, have the majority of votes, and in some instances because meetings are deemed quorate with one-third majority, three GPs out of the minimum membership of nine could make the final decisions (Smith *et al*, 1999).

Problems exist where minority views are less likely to succeed being thought less credible than the majority view, and if nurses are not well versed in macro-political skills they can be easily marginalised by the technical and medical-masculine method of decision making by GPs (Parkin, 1999b). Being in a minority also brings with it less opportunity to share the responsibilities board membership entails, and nurses are already finding that they have to spread themselves very thinly, to juggle PCG roles with existing posts (Sams and Boito, 1999). Nurse board members will require a great deal of vision, self-assurance and determination to triumph, as well as being able to present equality of knowledge in a language of certainty that promotes their position to one of equity on a level playing field. This type of person is the archetype of the ANP, who through expertise is not afraid to take risks or issue ultimatums. GPs remain extremely powerful in the configuration of PCG boards and this stems fundamentally from their united front and ability to mobilise quickly, advantages often unfamiliar to nurses. Because of this, nurses will have to overcome many organisational issues that medical colleagues do not, such as the election and selection process for boards. GPs have earned the right to be elected by their peers, whereas nurses have to face a two-tier selection system, having to overcome an initial nomination process and then interview by a health authority. There is a sharp contrast here, whereas GPs are not expected to meet competencies, satisfy hierarchy or justify their worth, ANPs as practice nurses will have to work hard to secure places, having to overcome a historical reputation of being task-orientated, medically focused and GP influenced (*Chapter 1*). A stereotype which may not be applied to trust-employed nurses.

The situation from the outside seems very idiosyncratic and there is little doubt that some practice nurses have done well at interviews, that many nurses experience no problem with collegial control and may even belong to a group who value their contribution. The reality is that for some it is not so easy and they are disappointed and disillusioned, there is a place here for ANPs to initiate change, lead the way and rise to the challenge.

Perspectives on ANPs as change agents

The future holds new opportunities in primary care, which depends inevitably on change and evolution to work in partnership and co-operation. Strategic change of this dimension can threaten core values and professional security, which can create barriers to innovation and progress. Nurses will need to change roles and identity — crossing over professional boundaries may create a culture of uncertainty, this shift can be inspiring or threatening (Williams and Sibbald, 1999). A move that challenges professional territories may force others to utilise power relations and political manoeuvres in order to dominate the change agenda on boards (Parkin, 1999c).

Success for ANPs working with PCGs or on PCG boards will depend therefore on their ability to effect changes through an understanding of organisations and change theory. Readers may find it useful to examine some of the change literature that is available in nursing. It is, however, the intention within this section to provide only an overview of how change agent skills are essential to advanced practice of the future, as well as to outline some pointers for ANPs to recognise or develop. It is also useful for others who may not wish to aspire to be ANPs, but just want to understand the principles of change and how to apply them, instead of remaining essentially a recipient.

The ability to facilitate change is not something ANPs will automatically possess, but everything begins somewhere and such expert nurses will already possess many positive attributes, which will help them. In change situations there is usually a need to influence key players and ANPs have many powers already. The main one of these is expert power, defined by Plant (1987) as:

> *Power from special knowledge which others need and do not possess. Respect for, and need for, this knowledge creates compliance.*

p. 44

ANPs reach this position and level of knowledge by reaching the pinnacle of their role, encompassing a level of expertise considered the penultimate but not the ultimate expression of proficiency (Pichert and Elam, 1985). This knowledge comes not from ideas of elitism, but from the ability and fortitude to constantly pursue and master facts and insight into a particular field or endeavour.

The resulting theoretical knowledge should stand ANPs in good stead in dealing with the persuasive scientific powers of many medical colleagues. ANPs also have vast experiential knowledge, which will be unique and thus sought after and valued. This source uses knowledge from a more holistic level which is thought different from logical intelligence and is fundamental to 'knowledge from the heart' (Katz, 1969). Handy (1985) sees disaster in concentrating on logical analytic intelligence and points out the value of other sources. The two most relevant in this instance are intra-personal intelligence, which is generated from knowing oneself and inner being, and interpersonal intelligence which is gained from ability to co-operate with and work through other people.

Realising that ANPs have something inherent to contribute can put them in a position of expert power that can challenge traditional ideas, prejudices and political manoeuvring. This confidence which comes from knowledge will be vital in helping to find problem-solving strategies and creative solutions. In managing change, the potential to produce constructive negotiation and mutual understanding is important — forcing expert power in an authoritarian manner is unlikely to work in PCGs. Facilitating participatory approaches and strategies are thought more likely to reduce resistance, produce greater acceptance, lead negotiation and be most effective within groups such as PCGs which serve the 'collective' interest (Parkin, 1999b).

Nurses, by the very fact they have been nominated onto boards, are in a powerful role and a source of power and influence. Throughout the literature, power is consistently linked to change.

Envisioning change is the dream of future nursing and therefore change agent skills will be essential for the ANP, if not for most nurses who wish to progress and become effective in ever-changing environments. Within the realms of practice Plant (1987) believes that everyone operates within a small central area of role, where safety comes from the low risk of surety of practice and position. Beyond this area is less secure because it encroaches on authority and confidence. The more people are able to extend into this sphere, the greater will be their circle of power, opportunity and choice. For nurses this will mean having the confidence and courage to embrace change themselves.

The ability to shape, grasp and utilise power will be vital in order to influence change successfully and to work effectively as a change agent. Plant (1987) identifies ten dimensions of role effectiveness which are useful for nurses to know in relation to either taking on new positions, wanting to initiate change or understand the positions they already find themselves in (*Table 6.1*)

The challenge of becoming successful in change requires competence and a disposition towards risk-taking. Assertiveness is an essential attribute to being a change agent as well as advanced practitioner. Traditionally, nurses have neither seen nor believed themselves to be assertive. This is historically a result of the dominance of medicine, seen to be more credible because of its scientifically-based knowledge and also its male superiority over a mainly female workforce. These factors have been reinforced and ingrained by previous nurse training and education. Nurses will have to adopt strategies to unlearn old behaviours, work to protect their own rights and trust their responses. This requires a person to be able to reflect on their relationship and behaviour with others and recognise their own biases, limitations, vulnerability and strengths.

Table 6.1: Ten dimensions of role effectiveness

1	Centrality	Role effectiveness will depend on the person feeling that their role is central to the organisation.
2	Integration	Role effectiveness is likely to be higher the more the role advances and utilises individual special strengths.
3	Proactivity	People respond to the expectations others have of their role, which provides individual satisfaction.
4	Creativity	Performance and effectiveness are higher in those who try new and unconventional ways of solving problems.
5	Connections	Effectiveness is increased if roles are connected to others and there is joint effort to understand problems.
6	Giving and receiving help	People have higher role effectiveness from opportunities to receive and give help.
7	Wider organisational value	Effectiveness is likely to be high if a person feels their role is likely to be of value.
8	Influence	The more influence a person exercises, the higher the role effectiveness.
9	Personal growth	Role effectiveness depends on the perception that the role facilitates opportunities to grow and develop.
10	Confronting problems	Finding solutions from confronting problems contributes to effectiveness.

Adapted from Plant, 1987

Risk-taking behaviour requires a quality of mind and a commitment to belief either individual or professional and is therefore not entered on lightly, reactively or without knowledge of the consequences and hope of the outcome. *Table 6.2* offers some useful ingredients in order to achieve strategies to aim for in bringing about change.

The ability to be resolute, think rationally and survive defeat if needs be differentiates the ANP from others.

Table 6.2: Ingredients for change
* Act early
* Identify patterns of thinking and shape them into a collective strategy
* Create a shared vision and awareness for change
* Listen actively
* Focus on 'what' and 'how'
* Move away from the past
* Communicate and be honest
* Turn perceived threats into opportunities
* Mobilise commitment
* Increase trust
* Utilise knowledge from the heart
* Monitor self within the situation and think rationally
* Be assertive and prepared to take risks
* Consider all possible outcomes
* Lead the way.

A willingness to take informed risk helps to initiate change as well as meet it. Change means the passing of one phase to another and Kurt Lewin (1951) has been most used by writers in understanding this process, and in introducing it he proposed three stages. Unfreezing (stage 1) which is breaking the habit in order to set the scene. This involves disturbing the equilibrium and creating discontent, which should establish motivation. Moving (stage 2) which is utilising new information to develop new ideas, feelings, behaviours and values. Refreezing (stage 3) which is recreating the new status quo, stabilising behaviour and maintaining the new change.

There are many ways to manage change and Jick (1993) suggests this is first, envisioning, as change has to be seen before anything can take place. Second, enabling, which is the unfolding of the process made from choices and third, implementation, which involves making the process happen. Change is not always this predictable though, yet the concepts are helpful and practitioners should never underestimate their powers, potential or ability to influence it.

The ANP as a leader

Community nursing seems set to change and practice nursing will be in the centre of this process. A window of opportunity exists to become a key performer alongside GPs. The nurses behind this change will need to initiate front-line provision of care facilitated by strong leadership. For practice nurses the ability to lead will be integral to move forward professionally and clinically; for ANPs, leadership is an essential competency to be developed or preserved. The concept of leadership, however, is not so straightforward and attempts to describe it are very indistinct and subjective. Despite this, there is never difficulty in recognising a good leader. Girvin (1998) has described such a person as a, 'Beacon in a murky world'. The search for recognition has led to several theories, and while these do not provide a definite answer, it is important that those who wish to take on leadership functions understand the principals used. It would be wrong to suggest that a theory on its own can define leadership or that effective leaders should adopt a particular one in isolation. It is suggested that potential leaders should adopt styles or a theory to best fit the situation.

The first theory sees leadership as integral to an individual personality or personal qualities and is know as the trait theory. Lists of traits appear in the literature, yet no traits seem common throughout suggesting that good leaders have different traits according to the circumstances. Most studies seem to single out the following:

- intelligence
- influence or dominance
- initiative
- self-confidence or self-assurance
- interpersonal skills
- inventiveness.

Handy (1985) also suggests the helicopter factor, which is the ability to rise above situations and view the situation in its entirety. In addition, Handy has noticed that successful leaders seem to have good health, be either above or well below average height or come from the upper socio-economic realms of society.

This personal quality approach as a stand-alone theory is much criticised as it is impossible to possess all the traits, and it is hard to see good leaders as only possessing certain characteristics and physical appearances. This issue stimulates further thinking that leadership implies a form of behaviour or specific activity, which gives rise to style theories.

This set of theories seems to refer to the authoritarian style, with power residing in control and punishment, and the democratic, fair styles, where power and responsibility is shared. Handy (1985) advocates that a supportive style leads to higher contentment and greater involvement. Style alone is still ambiguous in trying to provide conclusions to leadership that can be generalised, and the correct approach is also dependent on different situations or tasks. This notion gives rise to the third theory of leadership, the contingency theory.

The work of Fielder (1967) sheds more light onto contingency theory. He found that choice of style is dependent on the relationship with the group, the task to be done and the power of the leader within the organisation. This highlights the need for leaders to be flexible, and that importance often lies in getting the task done rather than in being democratic. This may be an important concept to explore in the light of recent PCG initiatives, as Parkin (1999a) believes, PCGs are high performance work teams working under a task culture.

Intrinsically linked to notions of leadership centring on the value of the task, are ideas of motivation. As Vroom (1964) illustrates, in order to influence followers groups must know how to accomplish the goals, be competent in doing so and at the same time, be able to achieve a degree of personal satisfaction.

Choice of style of leadership will also depend on a way of thinking about man and his management. Underlying assumptions exist about people that are often premeditated and these can colour views and actions. McGregor outlined two sets of assumptions about people in organisations, the Theory X and Theory Y, and understanding this concept can help to shed light onto the perspectives of leadership motivation. Within Theory X man is viewed by nature to be indolent, wanting to work as little as possible, resistant to change, lacking in any ambition, disliking responsibility and wanting to be led. Implications here are that in order to direct such individuals complete control is needed; efforts are manipulated through persuasion, reward or punishment. Theory Y is the opposite concept where people are seen as having potential for development and the capacity for responsibility. In contrast, people are treated positively and the notion is to facilitate individuals to realise their own goals and direct these and individual efforts towards objectives.

Man is complex and it may not be so realistic to divide motivations or assumptions about people into divided categories. However, the premise remains that reinforcing good behaviour can be more beneficial than punishment for unsatisfactory performance. What is evident is that choice of leadership will depend upon a set of values about people. Successful leadership has been linked to treating people by practising love (Harrison, 1987). This idea perhaps challenges other conventional ideas but is interwoven within the view that people should be directed from the heart in a way that feels right. This philosophy seems to integrate well into the intuitive nature of advanced practice and its expertise in knowing people (*Chapter 2*). Harrison advocates that to practice love in business, people need to be given credit for their ideas, which also need to be built on. People should be listened to empathetically and led to believe that their feelings have value, as well as always being trusted and given the benefit of the doubt. Each person is different and therefore valued for his or her uniqueness, which is to be nurtured and developed. This belief also incorporates giving help and assistance outside contractual arrangements and responsibilities of the job, to always look for the good and positive in others, which once found, should be acknowledged. While this applied initially to business relationships it is a philosophy that can be adopted in any leadership circumstances.

This strategy is not above risk, and it will take determination and belief for leaders to carry it through. But, as Harrison points out:

> *Perhaps, living in a competitive, abrasive and insecure world where relationships are often transitory and easily fractured, we are developing a hidden hunger to be loved a little bit.*

p. 17

This style of leadership would seem to illustrate the final theory of leadership, where it is an interactive, collaborative process, the group/relationship theory.

The complex relationship impinges on the leadership role as integral to that of mentorship and perhaps, because of the importance of the mentor role in advanced practice, it is worth deeper consideration. Like leadership, mentorship and mentoring is full of varied definitions and labels, understanding the influences and complexities however is vital if nurses wish to adopt a professional support relationship either in the workplace or in clinical teaching. Hart (1992) highlights the importance and challenge of helping individuals to make sense of their work needs and predicaments by asking questions, opening up new possibilities and letting go of the obsession to:

> *Merely build a quality workforce which will contribute to effectiveness. The incentive is to feel the pulse of these*

kinds of changes, to be a midwife to the unborn ideas, to articulate them and give them means of social expression which would make them conscious and actionable – this should be an educational task of primary importance.

p. 2000

Mentoring is, therefore, more than helping or guiding individuals, it is an enabling process in which the personal dimensions and characteristics of one person interact to influence, nurture and cultivate those of another into a dynamic relationship. It is relevant to point out that mentors do not have mystical powers, but expertise in directing individuals to use and discover their own talents in order to become successful in their own right. This process of facilitating potential, based on mutual magnetism and common interest, leads to reciprocal benefits of shared partnership. The relationship is different from other acquaintances, and common elements have been defined by Morton-Cooper and Palmer (2000). These are:

- the relationship is characterised by enabling and empowering
- the mentor is able to provide a repertoire of functions, such as helping, assisting and facilitating guidance while at the same time providing support. The mentor has to be an:
  - advisor
  - counsellor
  - coach
  - guide/networker
  - resource facilitator
  - role model
  - sponsor
  - teacher
- the role of the mentor comprises of interplay of personal, functional and relational aspects
- the individuals involved set mutual purposes and helper functions
- the individuals choose each other and the relationship has identifiable stages.

Leading through mentorship permeates all relationships within advanced practice, whether to help individuals grapple with the uncertainty of the workplace, to lead groups/individuals towards a common goal or vision, to fulfil a formal teaching role or a support system within clinical practice. Because mentoring is closely linked

to making the most of human potential this concept moves with the ANP into any professional role or sub-role they choose to undertake.
Like leadership, mentoring demands certain characteristics or attributes of the mentor and no one could aspire to all of these at one time. Ability will grow with experience if the person has sound qualities and a genuine desire to cultivate others. The following is a list of qualities that practitioners should eventually have in order to function as an effective mentor:

- interpersonal competence
- ability to help individuals self-evaluate and revise their picture of themselves
- be accepted as a role model, exemplifying characteristics associated with success in life and profession as well as a personality that merits imitation
- be committed to people and have a genuine interest in investing time into promoting their growth
- able to create a safe environment conducive for critical reflection and learning
- be capable of offering constructive feedback that allows individuals to be encouraged and able to learn from success or failure
- possess a network of valuable contacts and knowledge of resources
- able to motivate others, to challenge and encourage
- demonstrate imagination, patience, initiative and willingness to share understanding
- know human characteristics, personalities and feelings
- be reflective and able to think critically
- have a sense of humour.

Because of the very nature of friendship, the mentorship role, once established, may be a developing continuum or lifelong experience. Hunt and Michael (1983) outlined various stages that occur starting with 'initiation', then 'protégé', 'break up' and through to 'lasting friendship'. Whatever the duration of mentorship it is an intriguing process and a way to recover meaning in relationships and shared human experience.

Leadership, like mentoring, implies a passionate process, where change occurs not through management alone but through creating unity and a collective purpose with people. Koerner and Bunkers (1994) liken this to a spiritual process of:

Inner and outer realities being brought together in ways that assist individuals to integrate their unique inner world (values and beliefs) and outer world (life experience) into a unified whole.

p. 71

Leadership has many idiosyncrasies, and is also reliant upon individual personality; however, unlike mentorship it is dependent on the characteristics and attitudes of the followers, the environment and the task in hand. Because of its close links to groups and relationships with people it is often confused with authority and management theories, however, as pointed out by Malone (1996):

Leadership is at a higher development al level than management and that to be a leader, one inherently manages others.

p. 215

Leaders may also exercise authority but this is not essentially over people but within the interests of others. To become a leader is also implicitly linked to organisational culture, particularly as it is integral to the process of achieving shared values and objectives. To understand the culture of organisations is vital not only to promote leadership but also to comprehend individual working environments and backgrounds. It is also particularly relevant, as PCGs have been likened to virtual organisations. Handy (1985) offers some relevant organisational cultures seen in *Table 6.3*.

Northcott (2000) identifies five different cultures that some may find easier to recognise:

1. Personal pathology — where people are seen as making the mistakes and are sought out.
2. The bureaucratic culture — with laid down rules that prohibit innovation or individuality.
3. Watch-your-back culture — where departments or individuals are shown up.
4. Reactive/crisis driven — where attention is focused only on immediate concerns.
5. Learning/developmental — where growth, development and learning are encouraged.

Table 6.3: Relevant organisational cultures (reproduced with the permission of Charles Handy)			
	Power culture	**Role culture**	**Task culture**	**Person culture**
Visual picture	A spider's web	A Greek temple	A net	A galaxy of stars
Characteristics	A central control power source, with lines of power and influence radiating out from the middle. The spokes of these lines are connected by other specialist strands or power rings, which are the realms of activity and influence.	The organisation is a pediment resting on pillars of function or specialities.	This has threads of power aimed at getting the job done; some are thicker and stronger. Power lies in the interstices of the net at the knots.	This is a group of individuals where each one is the central point, with minimal structure in-between. Any structure is devised solely to serve the needs of individuals.
Source of power	Resource or personal power.	Position power.	Expert power.	Expert power (influence is shared). Personal power.
Mechanisms of control	Depends on trust with few rules and bureaucracy. Control exists in choosing and putting faith in the right people.	Strongly connected to bureaucracy because the work of the pillars is controlled by procedures and rules. This culture puts importance more on the job than the individual.	Seeks to bring together appropriate resources and the right people for the job, leaving them free to do it. Control lies in top management by means of allocation of projects, people and resource with no restriction.	Power base is shared with no management hierarchies. Organisation depends on individuals to exist.
Strengths	Organisations are usually strong, with the ability to move and respond quickly.	Offers security and predictability for those who want to climb up the pillars.	Very adaptable, individuals have a high degree of control over work, which fosters good working relationships and mutual respect.	Individuals are listened to, clear opportunities are listened to, clear opportunities and distribution of tasks and responsibilities.

Organisational culture is not always tangible, yet it is a controlling force in which people often sense whether they belong within it or not. In trying to understand culture it may be useful to identify the following within individual practices:

- the cultural artefacts, symbols, myths, rituals and routines
- the nature of the management, whether hierarchical or from shared influence
- the embedded values and beliefs, particularly in those who are the most influential
- the control mechanisms, whether directed by trust, monitoring or rules.

Leadership inevitably involves understanding organisational culture in order to be sensitive to its signals, the response of people and group reactions and expectations. It can be seen that successful leadership has many implications and major elements to be considered and understood, factors which lend themselves to subjectivity and misunderstanding. Yet future leaders need to be clear of the skills that they need to develop and practice from sound knowledge and vision of what the future will and should look like. This future seems more likely to take notice of nursing for within the wider political climate, the recent Government policy aims to promote nursing leadership, highlighted in the document *A Vision for The Future* (DoH, 1993b). There is now formal recognition given to the value of nursing input and opportunities to develop potential leaders.

Leadership in nursing now has the chance of success, and fundamental to this is the need to inspire vision based on collaboration and sharing. Visions do not come automatically. Future leaders will need foresight and the ability to seek relevant information to inform and develop a broad constructive picture. There is no guide to indicate which visions are right or wrong — individuals will need to trust their ideas. Within advanced practice this means utilising the essential charisma, intuition and instincts discussed in *Chapter 1*. Progressing the vision will also involve integrity and ANPs achieving goals through their multifaceted attributes and, above all, by creating credibility and inspiring confidence through acting as an example and actually living the values and beliefs.

The future leadership role in advanced practice will not only be to shape practice but also the political environment in which nursing functions. Antrobus (1998) highlights how:

Contemporary nursing leadership is concerned with influencing the political issues relevant to nursing and translating the impact of political changes into nursing practice.

p. 67

In order to gain understanding of the political arena, ANPs will need to read policies, become conversant with health and social agendas, network extensively and become involved and vocal in professional conferences and meetings. As Antrobus continues, leadership is open to everyone but particularly those operating at a clinical level and those able to think beyond nursing into understanding the position of the profession within the wider world of policy and politics.

Previously, nurses have not had much influence over policy, yet political ideology and policy substantially influence nursing. It would seem obvious that nurses, particularly ANPs, should be the ones to both direct their profession and influence the contextual reality in which they work and understand.

The politics for nursing cannot therefore be underestimated. Politics shapes nursing and therefore nursing leadership. To influence for nursing one needs to understand and influence the contextual ideology, which is shaped by the political.

Antrobus and Kitson, 1999, p. 753

New responsibilities and opportunities

ANPs need to be at the heart of nursing's future, operating as policy shapers and the grass root leaders of vision and clinical excellence. The potential to make this impact is not devoid of government incentive or reforms. The White Paper *A First Class Service: Quality in the new NHS* (DoH, 1998b) paved the way within the concept of clinical governance defined as, 'a framework through which NHS organisations are accountable for continuously improving the quality of their services and safeguarding high standards of care by creating an environment in which excellence in clinical care will flourish'. The Government agenda is for professionals to regulate themselves and be openly accountable in an attempt to prevent inequalities occurring within the NHS, brought about by differences in standards and commitments. The aim is to focus clear national frameworks with national standards.

The need to bring people together to regulate themselves is also reinforced in the document *Working Together: securing a quality workforce for the NHS* (DoH, 1998c) where it is stated, 'We must ensure that we have a quality workforce, in the right numbers, with the right skills and diversity, organised in the right way, to deliver the Government's service objectives for health and social care.'

PCGs will have a major role to play in promoting and providing clinical governance and this will be central to quality care. For the first time statutory duty places an obligation upon providers to guarantee satisfactory and responsive care that will be subject to outside scrutiny and review. A new structure, the National Institute of Clinical Excellence (NICE) is responsible for issuing guidelines on commissioning services and determining standards. PCGs are now accountable to the Commission for Health Improvement (CHIMP) which has wide-ranging powers to ensure that health professionals shape services and meet standards.

Opportunities exist to develop local initiatives and take clinical governance leads in practice. Nurses will be called upon to develop, deliver, maintain and monitor quality standards, all of which rely on experience, expertise and clinical excellence, the essential features of the ANP. The NHS E North Thames Regional Office (1998) identified several building blocks to achieving clinical governance: clinical audit, clinical effectiveness, clinical risk management, quality assurance and staff development. Practice nurses already have experience and knowledge of using clinical audit, quality assurance and achieving high quality patient care through implementation of guidelines within protocols for best practice. Practice nurses have also been involved in an element of risk management by learning from critical incidents and patient complaints in order to anticipate and present problems.

It seems that the way forward in meeting the remit for staff development for practice nurses is through clinical supervision, perhaps not such a familiar concept to general practice. During the past decade, practice nursing has developed because of its inherent freedom from nursing hierarchy and bureaucracy (*Chapter 1*), which at the same time has been a disadvantage because of the consequential lack of support by other nurses and possible isolation. Therefore, clinical supervision within practice nursing, unlike other nursing disciplines has not been well established in practice, and where it exists it has been sporadic and dependent upon individual initiatives of health authority practice nurse facilitators to secure money for pilot studies and projects. The need for support for practice nurses can be met by clinical supervision and the freedom from hierarchy that facilitated the opportunity to develop unrestricted can also be used to find the way to build up support systems. Clinical supervision has been described as:

> *A formal process of professional support and learning which enables individual practitioners to develop knowledge and competence, assume responsibility for their own practice and enhance consumer protection and safety of care in complex clinical situations.*

DoH, 1993

Minot and Adamski (1989) go on to state that it is a process where a practitioner reviews with a colleague their ongoing clinical work, relevant aspects and reactions to it.

Learning through support in the workplace is an essential process and the expert and experiential knowledge of the ANP makes their role of supervisor an obvious way forward for the future. This also seems more feasible as Minot and Adamski (1989) advocate that supervisors should be educated up to masters level in order to focus on theoretical and conceptual frameworks proficiently enough to bring about change and stimulate personal and clinical development.

It would be unworkable to say that only ANPs with a masters degree are capable of becoming supervisors. What is important is that the person, like an ANP, is able to relate theory to practice as Cairns (1998) states, 'Communicate effectively and offer philosophical but practical rationales based upon nursing values' (p. 24).

There should also be a genuine commitment and motivation to becoming a supervisor. As Rodriguez and Goorapah suggested (1998), there is no past evidence to indicate that supervision has come initially from nurses and as this is also coming from political incentive it may be viewed with suspicion, as power and control is being forced above and away from nursing. There is no reinforcement for clinical supervision, while it would seem reasonable to expect the UKCC to agree with supervision in principle, it would have little power to make it mandatory because of lack of finance and jurisdiction over employers involved, particularly in the case of GPs.

While there may be scepticism about adopting clinical supervision, it would be a shame to throw the baby out with the bath water, as it can be a way to meet the needs of clinical governance, provide support for isolated practice nurses and be an aid to their autonomy, as it would enhance practice, increase opportunity and widen perspectives and clinical views. Burnard (1990) also believes clinical supervision could actively resolve stress, by providing an environment in which nurses can re-establish separateness and a sense of detachment from patients and their lives.

It may seem relevant at this point to briefly explain what clinical supervision is, particularly as those wishing to establish it will need a sound theoretical underpinning. Proctor (1986) states that clinical supervision has three main functions:

- formative — which is developing skills and providing education
- restorative — which is to support
- normative — which involves quality control aspects of practice.

There is no general agreement as to how often supervisor and protégé should meet or the ideal length of time for each session. While vague this perhaps allows for flexibility in working and circumstances. Sessions themselves can take the form of case study, scenario or critical incident discussions. Houston (1990) outlines five types:

1. One to one with an expert from the same discipline.
2. One to one with a supervisor from a different discipline.
3. One to one peer supervision.
4. Group supervision — with or without external supervisor.
5. Network supervision — between those who do not work together every day.

Whatever the process chosen, Cutcliffe and Burns (1998) state that clinical supervision should be:

- enabling and supporting
- concerned with professional development
- client-centred
- an investment.

Clinical supervision is a complex process that calls for expertise in supervision; ultimately it is a way of informing practice and is an effective way to influence staff development and practice. To be able to motivate and inspire confidence is essential to effective supervision and professional development. Titchen (1998) likens the process to critical companionship, for which there are three conceptual domains: the relationship, rationality-intuitive and facilitative use of self-domain. Such theories suggest expertise and the ability to know oneself thoroughly, think critically, be able to bond and befriend others and transfer this craft and intimate knowledge into learning. The notion of clinical supervision, while discussed here in the light of the way forward in practice as well as a means to meeting clinical governance through quality care, cannot be considered without the mentorship and leadership implications mentioned earlier, and the aspirations of reflective practice discussed in *Chapter 5*.

Higher aspirations

The stage is set for more responsibilities for nurses in the future. Against this background of change is the possibility of new role development and aspirations for career development. Following the stance by the UKCC not to set standards for advanced practice the UKCC are pilot testing proposed standards and assessment processes for the award of a higher level of practice (UKCC, 1998). The standards for this have been devised around seven headings:

1. Providing effective healthcare.
2. Improving quality and health outcomes.
3. Evaluation and research.
4. Leading and developing practice.
5. Innovation and changing practice.
6. Developing self and others.
7. Working across professional and organisational boundaries.

Within these headings are a number of criteria which nurses need to meet in order to signify this level of practice. As can be seen by *Table 6.4.* these criteria match precisely the knowledge and skills of ANPs and particularly their role in general practice.

As a whole, the concept of advanced practice sits comfortably within the standards set for this higher level of practice (*Table 6.5*).

Table 6.4: The standard of higher level practice

Providing effective healthcare	Role of the ANP in general practice
* Create a climate in which patients and clients are empowered to make informed choices about their health and effective care.	* Direct access for patients * Utilise comprehensive consultation skills * Assesses from a background of knowing patients and families * Skilled in health provision.
* Receive direct referrals and undertake differential diagnosis using therapeutic communication, and valid, reliable and comprehensive patient and client-centred assessments which manage risk and are appropriate to needs, context and culture.	* Makes independent decisions in solving complex problems * Undertakes diagnosis of patient from comprehensive assessment skills, thinking and knowledge * Synthesis and analysis data from a high level * Experienced in audit and critical incident analysis.
* Prescribe therapeutic regimes, refer to other professions, order investigation, advise on changes in medication, and make appropriate decisions without recourse to other practitioners when in the interests of patients and clients.	* Autonomous and direct access role * Able to utilise protocol prescribing * High level of critical thinking skills * A highly visible practitioner, therefore has credibility and opportunities to network and refer to a wide range of professionals.
* Manage complete episodes of care and delegate aspects of care.	* Autonomous practitioner * May work with care assistants.
* In partnership with patients, clients and other professionals, make specific interventions informed by accepted best practice and appropriate to assessed needs, context and culture.	* High level of assessment skills which facilitate partnership in decision-making * Experienced in audit critical incident analysis * Carries out clinical supervision.

Table 6.5: Concept of advanced practice in relation to higher level of practice

Higher level practice headings	Role characteristics of an ANP	Achieved through
Providing effective health care. Improving quality and health outcomes Working across professional boundaries	Innovator Collaborator	Work in clinical governance Excellent interpersonal and problem-solving skills Potential or actual member of PCG Boards
Evaluation and research	Researcher	Utilises and develops research and audit Seeks money from awards and scholarships
Leading and developing practice	Leader Role model	Pioneering role
Innovation and changing practice	Change agent	Utilises political aware-ness and professional affiliations Innovative practice
Developing self and others	Mentor Educator	Undertakes clinical super-vision and supervisor role Public speaker

ANPs for the future will be required to register and provide evidence of achievement of these competencies. What is unclear at this stage is:

- how the UKCC intends to denote the mark of registration, whether by the suggested (H) suffix or not
- how often practitioners will be required to notify the UKCC of intention to continue to practice
- what exact evidence will be required, whether from reflective accounts, for example, or final oral assessment by a panel
- what, and if, a change should be made.

Hopefully the preliminary pilot testing that started in June 2000 on 300 practitioners will provide the answers and that this time the UKCC proposals will be more than rhetoric. Once this regulatory framework is established it may go some way in helping ANPs substantiate the role of consultant nurse, a post that will, 'provide an alternative career path for senior and experienced nurses who might otherwise enter management. The new posts will enable those nurses who want to advance their careers, but work to retain day to day contact' (NHS Executive, 1998).

Embarking on the future

The opportunity for professional growth and impact on patient health care delivery has never been more obtainable for nurses than at this present time. As individuals, ANPs need to believe in their own self-worth and that what they have to offer is marketable, valuable and the future of nursing. The way ahead lies in continuously pushing the boundaries and finding opportunities to be entrepreneurial and enact innovation (*Table 6.6*).

Table 6.6: Tactics for the future
* Attempt to gain knowledge of what is happening within your local area of practice
* Let go of insecurity to take advantage of new opportunities, which may feel uncertain
* Interact with people seen as role models and power players
* Be in contact with professionals who break new ground
* Join local communities and become active in professional organisations
* Position yourself to be seen, speak and write about what you know
* Become familiar with technology and communicate via the web
* Market yourself wherever possible with a well-developed CV and business cards.

Advanced practice will only survive in general practice if it is built upon a basis of sound partnership with GPs who do not see ANPs as a threat but as a valuable asset. This condition of respect will have to be earned by practitioners in showing through practice what it is they can do in a way that embraces a cost-conscious environment, and quality care that positively influences patient outcomes.

The ANP role must always be embedded in clinical expertise, incorporating the sub-role components as the environment lends itself, as Rolfe and Fulbrook (1998) explain:

> *You should not aim sometimes to be a practitioner, sometimes to be a teacher, sometimes to be a manager and sometimes to be a researcher; you should be a practitioner who sometimes teaches, sometimes manages and sometimes researches as part of your practice, as circumstances demand.*

p. 293

A key conviction will be to take courage and remain committed to keeping and promoting the title of advanced nurse practitioner, among the turbulence of professional inconsistencies and inadequacies. Predicting the future of advanced practice is not easy. The years ahead will almost certainly be stormy, but definitely exciting and the best role to be in. ANPs have the experience to take the lead in health care and turn their position into the visionary role it was originally meant to be. Some might say that this is a tall order for one person, but everything has to begin somewhere. All ANPs have to do is start.

References

Alfaro-LeFevre R (1995) *Critical Thinking in Nursing. A Practical Approach.* WB Saunders, Philadelphia

Altschul AT (1972) *Patient-Nurse Interaction. A Study of Interaction. Patterns in Acute Psychiatric Beds.* Churchill Livingstone, London

American Philosophical Association (1990) *Critical Thinking: A Statement of Expert Consensus for Purposes of Educational Assessment and Instruction: The Delphi Report: Research Findings and Recommendations Prepared for the Committee on Pre-college Philosophy.* American Philosophical Association, Millbrae CA

Anderson P (1995) Your role in prescribing. *Com Nurse* 1(11): 20–2

Antrobus S (1998) Thoroughly modern leaders. *Nurs Times* 94(18): 66–7

Antrobus S, Kitson A (1999) Nursing leadership: influencing and shaping health policy and nursing practice. *J Adv Nurs* 29(3): 746–53

Arons AB (1985) Critical thinking and the baccalaureate curriculum. *Liberal Educ* 71(2): 141–57

Arygle M (1978) *The Psychology of Interpersonal Behaviour.* 3rd edn. Penguin, Harmondsworth

Atkins S, Murphy K (1994) Reflective practice. *Nurs Stand* 8(39): 49–56

Bandman EL, Bandman B (1995) *Critical Thinking in Nursing.* 2nd edn. Appleton and Lange, Connecticut

Barnett v Chelsea and Kensington Hospital Management Committee [1969] 1 QB 428; [1968] 1 All ER 1068; [1968] 2 WLR 422

Barron AM (1989) The clinical nurse specialist as consultant. In Hameric AB, Spross JA (eds) *The Clinical Nurse Specialist in Theory and Practice.* 2nd edn. WB Saunders Company, Philadelphia

Benner P (1984) *From Novice to Expert. Excellence and Power in Clinical Nursing Practice.* Addison-Wesley Publishing, Menlo Park, CA

Benner P (1985) The oncology clinical nurse specialist as expert coach. *Oncology Nurse Forum* 12(2): 40–44

Benner P, Wrubel J (1989) *The Primacy of Caring.* Addison Wesley, New York

Benner P, Tanner C, Chisel C (1996) *Expertise in Nursing Practice, Caring, Clinical Judgement and Ethics.* Springer, New York

Benor R (1996) Therapeutic touch. *Br J Com Health Nurs* 1(4): 251–253

Beyer B (1984) Improving thinking-skills: defining the problem. *Phi Delta Kappan* 65: 486–90

Blake R, Mouton J (1983) *Consultation*. 2nd edn. Addison-Wesley Reading, Mass

Bolam v Friern Hospital Management Committee [1957] 1 WLR 582; [1957]1BMLR 1

Bowles N (1995) Story telling: a search for meaning within nursing practice. *Nurs Educ Today* **15**: 365–9

Bowling A (1981) *Delegation in General Practice. A Study of Doctors and Nurse.* Tavistock Publications, London

Brill N (1973) *Working with People.* JB Lippincott, New York

Brown J, Kitson A, McKnight T (1992) *Challenges in Caring. Explanations in Nursing and Ethics.* Chapman and Hall, London

Browning G (1982) *Updated ENT.* Butterworth Scientific, London

Bryan C (1995) Practice nursing: a study of the role. *Nurs Stand* **9**(17): 25–9

Burnard P (1990) *Learning Human Skills: An Experiential Guide for Nurses.* 2nd edn. Heinemann Nursing, Oxford

Cairns J (1998) Clinical supervision and the practice nurse. *J Com Nurs* **12**(20): 25

Calkin JD (1984) A model for advanced practice. *J Nurs Administration* **14**(1): 24–30

Caplan G (1970) *The Theory and Practice of Mental Health Consultation.* Basic Books, New York

Carper BA (1978) Fundamental patterns of knowing in nursing. *Adv Nurs Sci* **1**(1): 13–23

Carter R (1997) PNs: Facilitators of learning? *Pract Nurs* **8**(19): 14–16

Conway J (1998) Practising the art of reflection. *Pract Nurs* **9**(20): 15–19

Cooksley M (1995) Doctors' handmaidens. *Pract Nurs* **6**(2): 32–33

Cour J (1995) Screening for a solution. *Nurs Times* **91**(6): 40–2

Croft J (1980) Interviewing in physical therapy. *Physical Therapy* **16**: 1033–6

Cutcliffe J, Burns J (1998) Personal, professional and practice development: clinical supervision. *Br J Nurs* **7**(21): 1318–22

Damant M, Martin C, Openshaw S (1994) *Practice Nursing, Stability and Change.* Mosby Tavistock Square, London

Darbyshire P (1994) Skilled expert practice 'all in the mind'? A response to English's critique of Benner's novice to expert model. *J Adv Nurs* **19**: 755–61

Davies B (1995) Clarification of advanced nursing practice: characteristics and competencies. *Clinic Nurs Spec* **9**(3): 156–60

Department of Health and Social Security (1986) *Neighbourhood Nursing. A Focus for Care Report of the Community Nursing Review (Cumberledge Report).* HMSO, London

Department of Health (1987) *Promoting Better Health, Command No 249*. DoH, London

Department of Health (1989a) *Working for Patients*. HMSO, London

Department of Health (1989b) *General Practice in the National Health Service: The 1990 Contract*. DoH, London

Department of Health (1989c) *A Report on the Supply and Administration of Medicines under Group Protocols*. DoH, London: July

Department of Health (1989d) *Report on the Advisory Group on Nurses Prescribing*. DoH, London

Department of Health (1990) *Junior Doctors Hours: Heads of Agreement – Ministerial Group in Junior Doctor's Hours*. DoH, London

Department of Health (1993a) *Hospital doctors: Training for the Future, Report in the Working Group on Specialist Medical Training (The Calman Report)*. DoH, London

Department of Health and National Health Service Executive (1993b) *A Vision for the Future — the Nursing, Midwifery and Health Visiting Contribution to Health and Health Care*. DoH, London

Department of Health (1997) *The new NHS — modern, dependable*. Cmnd 3807. The Stationery Office, London

The Department of Health (1997) *The Extending Role of the Clinical Nurse. Legal implications and training requirements*. Health Circular (77) 22

Department of Health (1998a) *Clinical Examination of the Breast*. PL.CMO/98/1 DoH, London

Department of Health (1998b) *A First Class Service: Quality in the New NHS Health Services*. HMSO, London

Department of Health (1998c) *Working Together: Securing a Quality Workforce for the NHS*. HMSO, London

Department of Health (1999) *Review of Prescribing, Supply and Administration of Medicines: Final Report (Crown Report)*. DoH, London

Department of Health (2000) *The NHS Plan — A Plan for Investment. A Plan for Reform*. The Stationery Office, London

Descartes R (1984) The search for truth. In: Cottingham J, Stoothoff R, Murdoch D (eds) (1984) *The Philosophical Writings of Descartes*, Vol. 2. Cambridge University Press, Cambridge

Dimond B (1997) *Legal Aspects of Care in the Community*. Macmillian, Chippenham, Wiltshire

Donaldson R, Donaldson L (1983) *Essential Community Medicine*. MTP Press Ltd, Lancaster

Donoghue v Stevenson [1932] AC 562; [1932] 1 All ER 1

Dreyfus HL, Dreyfus SE (1986) *Mind over Machine: The Power of Human Intuition and Expertise in the Era of the Computer.* Free Press, New York

Dunn B (1993) Use of therapeutic humour by psychiatric nurses. *Br J Nurs* **2**(9): 468–73

Edwards S (1998) Critical thinking and analysis: a model for written assignments. *Br J Nurs* **7**(3): 159–66

Ekman P, Frieson WV (1972) Hand movements. *J Communication* **22**: 253–374

Emden C (1991) Becoming a reflective practitioner. In: Gray G, Pratt R (eds) (1991) *Towards a Discipline of Nursing.* Churchill Livingstone, Melbourne

Ennis EA (1985) A logical basis for measuring critical thinking skills. *Educational Leadership* **42**: 45–8

Facione NC, Facione PA (1994) *Holistic Critical Thinking Scoring Rubric.* The California Academic Press, Millbrae, California

Fawcett J (1984) *Analysis and Evaluation of Conceptual Models of Nursing.* FA Davis, Philadelphia

Fenton MU (1985) Identifying competencies of clinical nurse specialists. *J Nurs Admin* **15**(12): 31–7

Fernandez E (1997) Just 'doing the observations' reflective practice in nursing. *Br J Nurs* **6**(16): 939–43

Fielder FE (1967) *A Contingency Theory of Leadership and Effectiveness.* McGraw-Hill, London

Frost S (1998) Perspectives in advanced practice: an educationist's view. In: Rolfe G, Faulbrook P (eds) *Advanced Nursing Practice.* Butterworth-Heinmann, Oxford: 33

Fulbrook P (1998) Advanced practice: the 'advanced practitioner' perspective. In: Rolfe G, Fulbrook P (eds) *Advanced Nursing Practice.* Butterworth-Heinmann, Oxford

Garver E (1986) Critical thinking: them and us. A response to Arnold Aron's critical thinking and the baccalaureate curriculum. *Liberal Education* **72**: 245–52

General Medical Services Committee (1986) *Report to the Special Conference of Representatives of Local Medical Committees.* British Medical Association, General Medical Services Committee, London

Gibbs G (1988) *Learning by Doing: A guide to teaching and learning methods.* Further Education Unit, Oxford Brookes University, Oxford

Gillion R (1986) *Philosophical Medical Ethics.* Wiley, Chichester

Girvin J (1998) *Leadership and Nursing.* Macmillan Press Ltd, London

Grundstein-Amado R (1992) Differences in ethical decision-making processes among nurses and doctors. *J Adv Nurs* **17**: 129–37

Hagell E (1988) Nursing knowledge: women's knowledge. A sociological perspective. *J Adv Nurs* **14**: 226–233

Halpern DF (1989) *Thought and Knowledge: An Introduction to Critical Thinking.* 2nd edn. Lawrence Erlbaum Associates, New Jersey

Hampton D (1994) Expertise: The true essence of nursing art. *Adv Nurs Sci* **17**(1): 15–24

Handy C (1985) *Understanding Organisations.* Penguin Books, Middlesex

Hardy R (1995) Practice nursing in partnership. *Pract Nurs* **6**(6): 30–2

Harrison R (1987) *Organization Culture and Quality of Service: a strategy for releasing love in the workplace.* Association for Management Education and Development, London

Hart MU (1992) *Working and Educating for Life.* Routledge, London

Hawkins JW (2000) Caring for all: an old idea for a new millennium. *Clinical Excellence for Nurse Practitioners* **4**(3): 131–2

Health Service Journal (1997) Papering over the cracks? *Health Service Journal* Dec: 17

Heath H (1998) Reflection and patterns of knowing in nursing. *J Adv Nurs* **27**: 1054–9

Heron J (1990) *Helping the Client. A Creative Practical Guide.* Sage Publications, London

House of Commons (1998) The NHS White Papers — Research Paper. 98/15, House of Commons

Houston G (1990) *Supervision and Counselling.* The Rochester Foundation, London

Hunt D, Michael C (1983) Mentorship — a career training development tool. *Academy of Management Review* **3**: 457–85

Hyde V (1997) Community practice teachers. *Pract Nurs* **8**(20): 16–18

Jameton A (1984) *Nursing Practice: the Ethical Issues.* Prentice-Hall, Englewood Cliffs NJ

Jick TD (1993) *Managing Change: Cases and Concepts.* Irwin, Burr Ridge IL

Johns C (1994) Nuances of reflection. *J Clin Nurs* **3**: 71–5

Jones SA, Brown L (1991) Critical thinking: impact of nursing education. *J Adv Nurs* **16**: 529–33

Kahn RL, Connell CF (1957) *The Dynamics of Interviewing.* Wiley, New York

Katz FE (1969) Nurses. In: Etzioni A (ed) *The Semi-Professions and Their Organisation: Teachers, Nursing, Social Workers.* The Free Press, New York

Keenan J (1999) A concept analysis of autonomy. *J Adv Pract* **29**(3): 556–62

King RC (1983) Refining your assessment techniques. *RN* **46**: 43–7

Koerner J, Bunkers S (1994) Transformational leadership: The power of symbol. In: Hein E, Nicholson MJ eds *Contemporary Leadership Behaviour*. 4th edn. JB Lippincott, Philadelphia

Landis RE, Michael WB (1981) The factorial validity of three measures of critical thinking within the context of Guilfords Structure of Intellect Model for a sample of ninth grade students. *Educational and Psychological Measurement* **41**: 1147–66

Larson KM, Smith CK (1981) Assessment of nonverbal communication in the patient physician interview. *J Fam Pract* **12**(3): 481–8

Lewin K (1951) *Field Theory in Social Science*. Harper and Row, New York

Lilley R (1999) Bespoke primary care. *Pract Nurs* **10**(7): 6

Major B (1981) Gender patterns in teaching behaviour. In: Mayo C, Henley NM (eds) *Gender and Non-verbal Behaviour*. Springer-Verlag, New York

Malone B (1996) Clinical and professional leadership. In Hamric A, Spross J, HansonC (eds) *Advanced Nursing Practice. An Integrative Approach*. WB Saunders Company, Philadelphia

Marsh GN, Dawes ML (1995) Establishing a minor illness nurse in a busy general practice. *Br Med J* **310**: 778–80

May V (1997) Nurse's readiness to prescribe. *Comm Nurs* Special News Report, September: 8–9

McCartney M, Tyrer S, Brazier M, Prayle D (1999) Nurse prescribing radicalism or tokenism? *J Adv Nurs* **29**(2): 348–54

McClure L (1995) Community nurses and carers: what price support and partnership? In: Cain P, Hyde V, Hawkins E (eds) *Community Nursing: Dimensions and Dilemmas*. Arnold, London

McCormack B (1993) How to promote quality of care and preserve patient autonomy. *Br J Nurs* **26**: 338–41

McPeck J E (1981) *Critical Thinking and Education*. Martin Robertson, Oxford

Mead M (1992) Health Promotion. Gazing into the crystal ball. *Pract Nurs* **5**(3): 173

Mill J S (1910) *Utilitarianism, Liberty and Representative Government*. JM Dent

Minot S, Adamski TJ (1989) Elements of effective clinical supervision. *Perspectives in Psychiatric Care* **25**(2): 22–6

Morton-Cooper A, Palmer A (2000) *Mentoring Preceptorship and Clinical Supervision: A Guide to Professional Roles in Clinical Practice*. 2nd edn. Blackwell Science, Oxford

Munhall P (1993) 'Unknowing': towards another pattern of knowing in nursing. *Nursing Outlook* **41**(3):12–8

Neighbour R (1987) *On having two heads. The Inner Consultation.* MTP Press Limited, London: 51–63

NHS Executive (1996) *Clinical Guidelines: Using Clinical Guidelines to Improve Patient Care within the NHS.* DoH, London

NHS Executive (1998) *Nurse Consultants.* (HSC, 1998/161) 22 September, DoH, London

NHS ME (1991) *Junior Doctors: The New Deal.* NHS ME, London

NHSE North Thames Regional Office (1998) *Clinical Governance in North Thames: A Paper for Discussion and Consultation.* June 1998, Department of Public Health, London

Nolan M, Lindh U, Tishelman C (1998) Nursing's knowledge base: does it have to be unique? *Br J Nurs* **7**(5): 270–6

Northcott N (2000) Clinical supervision – professional development or management control? In: Spouse J Redfern L (eds) *Successful Supervision in Health Care Practice. Promoting Professional Development.* Blackwell Science, Oxford

O'Connor N (2000) Use of patient group directions in England is ratified in law. *Primary Health Care* **10**(71): 7

O'Hara Deveraux M (1991) Nurse practitioners in North America. In: Salvage J (ed) *Nurse Practitioners: Working for Change in Primary Health Care Nursing.* King's Fund Centre, London

Olson J (1995) Empathy and patient distress. *Image* **27**: 317–32

Paniagua H (1998) The US experience of advanced practice. *Pract Nurs* **19**(19): 8–11

Paniagua H (1995) The scope of advanced practice: action potential for practice nurses. *Br J Nurs* **4**(5): 269–74

Paniagua H (1997) Consultations: In practice. *Pract Nurs* **8**(8): 20–2

Parkin P (1999a) Managing change in the community 1: the case of PCGs. *Br J Nurs* **4**(1): 19–27

Parkin P (1999b) Managing change in the community 2: partnership in PCGs. *Br J Nurs* **4**(4): 188–95

Parkin P (1999c) Managing change in the community 3: conflict in PCGs *Br J Nurs* **4**(6): 275–82

Partridge E (1957) *Usage and Abusage.* 5th edn. Penguin, Aylesbury

Pease A (1985) *Body Language.* Sheldon Press, London

Pichert J, Elam P (1985) Differences between novices and experts. *Diabetes Educator* **11**: 9–12

Plant R (1987) *Managing Change and Making it Stick.* Fontana. An imprint of Harper Collins Publishers, London

Poole J (1999) Taking responsibility for our future. *Pract Nurs* **10**(14): 20

Prince E (1999) Unpublished assignment on Advanced Health Assessment For Health Professionals for the MSc in Advanced Clinical Practice for the University of Wolverhampton

Proctor B (1986) Supervision: a co-operative exercise in accountability. In: Marken M, Payne M (eds) *Enabling and Ensuring*. Leicester National Youth and Community Work, Leicester

Reedy BLEC (1972) *Organisation and Management; The General Practice Nurse*. Update 5: 75–78

Reigle J (1996) Ethical decision-making skills. In: Hamric A, Spross J, Hanson C (eds) *Advanced Nursing Practice. An Integrated Approach*. WB Saunders Company, London

Reily BJ, Di-Angelo JA Jr (1990) Communication: a cultural system of meaning and value. *Human Relations* **43**(2): 129–14

Reveley S (1998) The role of the triage Nurse Practitioner in general medical practice: an analysis of the role. *J Adv Nurs* **28**(3): 584–91

Reveley S, Money B (1998) Practice-based education: the nurse practitioner in primary care. *Br J Nurs* **3**(5): 226–32

Riev S (1994) Error and trial; the extended role dilemma. *Br J Nurs* **3**(4): 168–174

Robinson JA (1994) Problems with paradigms in a caring profession. In: Smith J (ed) *Models, Theories and Concepts*. Blackwell Scientific, London

Rodriguez P, Goorapah D (1998) Clinical Supervision for nurse teachers: the pertinent issues. *Br J Nurs* **7**(11): 663–74

Rolfe G (1997) Science, abduction and the fuzzy nurse an exploration of expertise. *J Adv Nurs* **25**: 1070–5

Rolf G (1998) Beyond expertise: reflective and reflexive nursing practice. In: Johns C, Freshwater D (eds) *Transforming Nursing through Reflective Practice*. Blackwell Science, Oxford

Rolfe G, Fulbrook P (1998) *Advanced Nursing Practice*. Butterworth-Heinmann, Oxford

Rowden R (1984) Doctors can work with the nursing process: a reply to Professor Mitchell. *Br Med J* **288**: 216–19

Royal College of Nursing and Royal College of General Practitioners (1974) *Report of the Joint Working Party in Nursing in General Practice in the Reorganised National Health Service*. RCN, London

Royal College of Nursing (1993) *Protocols and Nursing: Guidance for Good Practice. RCN Issues in Nursing Series. 21*. RCN, London

Royal College of Nursing (1996) *Family Planning and Contraception in General Practice: Guidance for Nurses. RCN Issues in Nursing Series 41*. RCN, London

Royal College of Nursing (1997) *Factsheet 2. Extension of prescribing powers to nurses.* RCN, London

Salussolia M (1997) Is advanced nursing practice a post or a person? *Br J Nurs* **6**(16): 928–33

Sams D, Boito H (1999) Taken on board. *Nurs Times* **95**(13): 56–7

Schaefer J (1974) The interrelatedness of the decision-making process and the nursing process. *Am J Nurs* **74**(10): 1852–5

Schein EH (1969) *Process Consultation: Its Role in Organisational Development.* Addison-Wesley, Reading, Mass

Schön D (1983) T*he Reflective Practitioner; How Professionals Think in Action.* Basic Books, New York

Scott RS (1985) When it isn't life or death. *Am J Nurs* **85**(1): 19–20

Sharp JF, Wilson JA, Ross L, Barr-Hamilton RM (1990) Ear wax removal: a survey of current practice. *Br Med J* **301**: 251–3

Smith K, Dickson M, Sheof R (1999) Second among equals. *Nurs Times* **95**(13): 54–55

Smith M (1994) Practice nursing professional occupation. In: Luft S, Smith M (eds) *Nursing in General Practice.* Chapman and Hall, London

Smith M (1995) The core of advanced practice nursing. *Nurs Sci Q* **8**(1): 2–3

Stern K (1995) Clinical guidelines and negligence liability. In: Deighan M, Hitch S (eds) *Clinical Effectiveness: From Guidelines to Cost-Effective Practice.* Earlybrave Publications Ltd, Brentwood

Styles M (1996) Conceptualisations of advanced nursing practice. In: Hamric A, Spross J, Hanson C (eds) *Advanced Nursing Practice. An Integrated Approach.* WB Saunders Company, London

Sutton F, Smith C (1995) Advanced nursing practice: new ideas and new perspectives. *J Adv Nurs* **21**: 1037–4

Synder M (1995) Professional Communication: publishing and public speaking. In: Synder M, Mirr M (eds) *Advanced Practice Nursing: A Guide to Professional Development.* Springer Publishing Company, New York

Tanner C, Benner P, Chelsea C, Gordon D (1993) The phenomenology of knowing the patient. *Image* **25**: 237–80

Thompson CG, Ryan SA, Kitzman H (1990) Expertise: the basis for expert system development. *Adv Nurs Sci* **13**(2): 1–10

Thompson J (1988) Communicating with patients. In: Fitzpatrick R, Hinton J, Newman S, Scambler G, Thompson J (eds) *The Experience of Illness.* Tavistock Publications, London

Titchen A (1998) *A Conceptual Framework for Facilitating Learning in Clinical Practice.* Occasional Paper No 2, Radcliffe Infirmary, Royal College of Nursing Institute, Oxford

Touché Ross (1994) *Evaluation of Nurse Practitioner Pilot Projects.* South East Thames Regional Health Authority. Touché Ross Management Consultants

Tschudin V (1992) *Ethics in Nursing. The Caring Relationship.* Butterworth Heineman Ltd, Oxford

Tunnadine P (1992) *Insights into Troubled Sexuality. A Case Profile Anthology.* Revised edn. Chapman and Hall, London

Turnball J (1999) Intuition in nursing relationships: the result of 'skills' or 'qualities'? *Br J Nurs* **18**(5): 302–6

United Kingdom Central Council for Nursing, Midwifery and Health Visiting (1990) *The Report of the Post Registration Education and Practice Project.* UKCC, London

United Kingdom Central Council for Nursing, Midwifery and Health Visiting (1992a) *The Scope of Professional Practice.* UKCC, London

United Kingdom Central Council for Nursing, Midwifery and Health Visiting (1992b) *The Code of Professional Practice.* UKCC, London

United Kingdom Central Council for Nursing, Midwifery and Health Visiting (1994) *The Future of Professional Practice – the Council's Standards for Education and Practice Following Registration.* UKCC, London

United Kingdom Central Council for Nursing, Midwifery and Health Visiting (1995) *PREP and You.* UKCC, London

United Kingdom Central Council for Nursing, Midwifery and Health Visiting (1996) *The Council's Standards for Education and Practice following Registration (PREP). Transitional Arrangements — Specialist Practitioner Title/Specialist Qualification. Position Statement.* UKCC, London

United Kingdom Central Council for Nursing, Midwifery and Health Visiting (1997) *PREP — the nature of advanced practice. Cc/97/06.* UKCC, London

United Kingdom Central Council for Nursing, Midwifery and Health Visiting (1998) *A Higher Level of Practice — Consultation Document. Register 24. 10.* UKCC, London

United Kingdom Central Council for Nursing, Midwifery and Health Visiting (1999) *A Higher Level of Practice. Report of the UKCC's Proposal for a Revised Regulatory Framework for Post-Registration Clinical Practice.* UKCC, London

Van Manen M (1990) *Researching Lived Experience: Human Science for an Action Sensitive Pedagogy.* Althouse Press, Toronto

Van Manen M (1991) *The Tact of Teaching: The Meaning of Pedagogical Thoughtfulness*. State University of New York Press, New York

Vroom V (1964) *Work and Motivation*. John Wiley, London

Walker R (1995a) Breast examination. *Pract Nurs* **6**(16): 19

Walker R (1995b) Cardiology. *Pract Nurs* **6**(14): 15

Walsh M (1999) Nurses and nurse practitioners: priorities in care. *Nurs Stand* **13**(24): 38–42

Watson G, Glaser EM (1991) *Critical Thinking Appraisal Manual*. Psychological Corporation, Kent

Wedderbum Tate C (1997) Nurse 2000. *Nurs Stand* **12**(1): 24

Williams A, Sibbald B (1999) Changing roles and identities in primary health care: exploring a culture of uncertainty. *J Adv Nurs* **29**(3): 737–45

Wilson JMG, Jungner RG (1968) *Principles and Practice of Screening for Disease. Public Health Paper 34*. WHO, Geneva

Woods L (1997) Conceptualising advanced nursing practice, curriculum issues to consider in the educational preparation of the advanced practice nurse in the UK. *J Adv Nurs* **25**: 820–8

Index